Recovery after Rehab

Recovery after Rehab

A Guide for the Newly Sober and Their Loved Ones

Joseph Nowinski

ROWMAN & LITTLEFIELD
Lanham · Boulder · New York · London

Published by Rowman & Littlefield
An imprint of The Rowman & Littlefield Publishing Group, Inc.
4501 Forbes Boulevard, Suite 200, Lanham, Maryland 20706
www.rowman.com

6 Tinworth Street, London SE11 5AL, United Kingdom

British Library Cataloguing in Publication Information Available

Library of Congress Cataloging-in-Publication Data

Names: Nowinski, Joseph, author.
Title: Recovery after rehab : a guide for the newly sober and their loved ones / Joseph Nowinski.
Description: Lanham : Rowman & Littlefield, [2020] | Includes bibliographical references and index. | Summary: "This book picks up where 'rehab' leaves off, and where the real work of recovery from substance abuse begins. It is a practical guide not only for the newly sober, but for their loved ones as well" — Provided by publisher.
Identifiers: LCCN 2020047773 (print) | LCCN 2020047774 (ebook) | ISBN 9781538142523 (cloth) | ISBN 9781538142530 (epub)
Subjects: LCSH: Substance abuse—Treatment. | Addicts—Rehabilitation. | Recovering addicts.
Classification: LCC RC564 .N688 2020 (print) | LCC RC564 (ebook) | DDC 362.29—dc23
LC record available at https://lccn.loc.gov/2020047773
LC ebook record available at https://lccn.loc.gov/2020047774

For Becca, Greg, and Maggie
So proud to have you as my kids

Contents

Introduction

Point of Departure

The term "point of departure," originally a nautical term, is defined as "the precise location of a vessel, established in order to set a course, especially in beginning a voyage in open water."[1]

There is probably no better analogy—and no better starting point—for the subject of this book than this idea of a point of departure. Recovery from any severe substance-use disorder (or any addiction for that matter) is indeed best thought of as a journey across open water. In this case it begins with formal treatment of one kind or another. For many of those faced with such disorders, as well as those who love them, this step typically marks a crossroads and is met with relief and with hope for a better future. That said, treatment (or rehab) is not an end point; rather, it marks the starting point for this voyage. As many who have relapsed can attest, success is far from guaranteed.

This book will examine those factors that can enhance the chances of success of the voyage into recovery as well as those that can sabotage it. It takes the position that recovery is best thought of not as a sole voyage across open and often perilous waters but rather as a journey that is best taken collaboratively between a newly sober man or woman and his or her loved ones. In that sense it is a departure from the common advice to let the newly sober person take sole responsibility for recovery while loved ones merely look on and take care of themselves. Such advice is frequently frustrating and unsatisfying to loved ones. Similarly, dated concepts like "enabling" and "codependence" have evolved into pejorative terms that tend to pathologize loved ones, leading to shame and further frustration. We will redefine these terms here to clarify their true meaning and thereby free loved ones to become true partners in the recovery process.

We will begin with a brief look at treatment and rehab and what loved ones and those with substance-use disorders can reasonably expect. Then, with this as our point of departure, we shove off into open water.

Auspicious Beginnings

The Pink Cloud

The term "pink cloud" was traditionally (and in some quarters still is) used within the recovery community to refer to the emotional and cognitive state that the substance abuser experiences once he or she has detoxed from and is free (perhaps for the first time in many years) from enslavement to alcohol or other drugs. Today, in our age of opioid dependence, that new freedom may require substituting prescribed medication for heroin or prescription opioids, at least for a time.

In effect, the newly detoxed and sober individual feels great—hence the "pink cloud." They often report that their mind is clear and their body feels "normal" for the first time in years. But there is a potential trap here, namely, believing that they are "cured" and also that their loved ones will share their newly found happiness. But this is not always the case. Several factors can contribute to this. First, ambivalence may more accurately describe the emotional state of loved ones at this point. True, they may be relieved that their loved one finally entered treatment; and they may be happy that the newly sober loved one feels good. At the same time, they are apt to be wary and cautious or, as one partner put it, "drained to the point of exhaustion, and hard to feel excited."

This discrepancy between what the newly detoxed family member and his or her loved ones is experiencing can lead to disappointment and frustration when the sober substance-user returns home. Here is an example.

"I finally agreed to enter rehab after I got a DUI and also after my supervising partner unexpectedly walked into my office and smelled the smoke from the joint I foolishly tried to sneak." Tyler, a forty-year-old attorney, explained that he'd been drinking alcohol pretty much daily since his late teens and smoking pot most days after work for the past decade. About a year earlier he'd also started using on weekends cocaine that he obtained through a client with connections in the restaurant business. Although he was able to maintain a demanding workload at the law firm, he admitted that his home life had been a different story. His routine was to get home from the office, have a few drinks before dinner, and then retreat to his "home office" where he would smoke some weed and watch the news until he'd fall asleep, typically by nine. He admitted that his daily interactions with his wife and nine-year-old daughter would most often total no more than twenty minutes of his daily schedule. Meanwhile, it was his wife who took their daughter to her gymnastics classes, soccer games, and doctor appointments, who attended school parent meetings, and so on.

> I spent thirty days in rehab and once I got through detox I couldn't believe how good I felt. I spoke with my wife briefly every evening, but the policy at the rehab was that these could be ten-minute calls, max. I have a daughter, but I didn't talk with her for more than a few minutes while I was in rehab.
>
> My wife picked me up at the airport after I was discharged. I remember she gave me a quick hug and asked me how the flight was, but otherwise we spoke little on the drive home. I was feeling good and looking forward to being home. I don't know exactly what I was expecting—a Mariachi band on the front porch? A block party with fireworks? But what I actually got was nothing much. My daughter wasn't even home when I got there. She was at a friend's, and she hardly had time to say hello when she got dropped off and retreated to her room. It was pretty deflating, to tell the truth.

What accounts for situations like this? For one thing, as the addict's "relationship" with substance use grows stronger and comes to take a prominent role in his or her lifestyle, other relationships (marriage, children, friendships, colleagues, and coworkers) progressively fade into the background. Understandably this can set the stage for anger, resentment, and alienation that can undermine the real recovery journey that begins *after* rehab. Such reactions as these on the part of loved ones are rarely addressed either in treatment or after.

THE OPAQUE REHAB INDUSTRY

A second factor contributing to ambivalence on the part of loved ones is that rehab is too often opaque, and that is a problem. Almost everyone is familiar with the scene in *The Wizard of Oz* where Toto, Dorothy's dog, pulls back the curtain to reveal the secret behind the powerful wizard, who turns out to be no wizard after all. Unfortunately, for many loved ones of those who enter rehab for addiction, the rehab center itself can seem very much like that curtain—only they hope there is really a wizard inside! They may look to rehab as the solution to their dilemma yet know very little to nothing about what actually goes on behind closed doors. And some rehabs advertise services that sound more like a vacation than treatment. So although the newly sober individual may be feeling on top of the world and confident, their loved ones again are apt to be uninformed and understandably wary.

This opaque quality of substance abuse treatment sets it apart from other forms of medical treatment. For most forms of medical and mental health treatment, there are established procedures and interventions for assessing and dealing with them. Diabetes, high cholesterol, and hypertension, for example, are typically diagnosed in the same ways and dealt with via specified treatment options. A diagnosis of cancer typically draws in the entire family of the patient, who are included in discussions, including prognosis and treatment options. And family members continue to be included with regard to progress and further treatment if necessary.

The same is pretty much true for mental health disorders such as severe depression, social anxiety, and bipolar disorder. Of course, there is some latitude afforded to the professional doing the treatment, but by and large, third-party payers such as insurance carriers will only pay for diagnosis and treatment if it falls within established parameters. In this way loved ones can be brought into the picture so as to understand the problem as well as how it is being tackled.

The above is not at all the case when it comes to addiction treatment. At this time there are still no established standards for treating substance-use disorders. There are, in fact, what are called evidence-based treatments for use disorders. These treatments have been tested through rigorous research and deemed to be effective. Descriptions of them can be found by visiting www.drugabuse.gov or simply Googling "evidence-based practice for substance-use disorders." I would encourage the loved ones of those entering rehab to visit these resources.

Although evidence-based treatments (based, in other words, on sound clinical research) do exist, there are currently no requirements that treatment centers use them nor is there any system in place to monitor these agencies' practices. In other words, substance abuse rehab is currently an unregulated industry. This accounts for a wide diversity in terms of what actually goes on inside any particular rehab center.

According to the National Survey of Substance Abuse Treatment Service (N-SSATS), as of 2017 there were 13,585 substance abuse treatment facilities in the United States serving 1,356,015 clients.[1] These numbers included individuals in a variety of treatment settings ranging from inpatient or residential to intensive outpatient (typically several hours a day over several days a week) to weekly outpatient treatment. Today the greatest number of treatment facilities offer treatment for both alcohol and drug abuse (usually concurrent). The trend—driven largely by cost—is toward shorter residential treatment in favor of intensive outpatient care. As a loved one, you may expect this to be the treatment proposed for the substance abuser.

Despite the lack of standardization, the substance abuser and his or her loved ones alike are left to assume that what goes on in treatment is actually relevant to recovery from alcohol or drug abuse. Understandably, being essentially blind to the actual content and process of treatment for a substance-use disorder is another factor that may contribute to some ambivalence as opposed to full-throated confidence on the part of loved ones.

RELAPSE

Another factor that contributes to ambivalence on the part of loved ones of the newly sober is the reality of relapse. It's no secret that the record of a successful open-water crossing starting from the point of departure that is rehab is—to put it mildly—less than stellar.

As optimistic as the loved ones of the newly sober individual may wish to be, the reality of potential relapse typically lurks in the background of consciousness, and it should not be swept under the carpet. This is not to question the intentions of the individual leaving treatment so much as it is to recognize that good intentions do not always translate into positive outcomes. The National Institute on Drug Abuse (NIDA), for example, cites a 40–60 percent chance of relapse from a substance-use disorder.[2] While this statistic may seem discouraging, it's important to keep in mind that NIDA points out that the relapse rate for people treated for diabetes is in the 30–50 percent range, and for hypertension it is in the 50–70 percent range. Does this mean that these treatments are not effective? No. It means that many patients fail to follow through consistently with treatment following initial diagnosis and treatment. In short, their journeys go awry after their point of departure.

A COLLABORATIVE APPROACH

The goal of this book—which is aimed at both the newly sober man or woman and his or her loved ones—is to provide a guide to how they can (and should) approach recovery from a substance-use disorder collaboratively. They are each equal stakeholders in the long-term outcome for the newly sober, his or her partner, and the larger family. Substance abuse affects all of these individuals; therefore, recovery should not rightly leave out any of them. It is true that the recovering person must shoulder much of the responsibility for following through after treatment, but transparency, support, and communication also have their place in assuring a safe journey.

What follows is a guide to how recovery can be strengthened, particularly through the first year following treatment, which is critical. To begin, the newly sober individual and his or her loved ones should read the above material and discuss it. How much can you relate to the ideas and facts presented here? What were your expectations at the time the substance abuser entered treatment? What are your greatest concerns now? Finally, does the idea of being collaborators—co-equal stakeholders—in recovery sound like a good idea, and one worth pursuing?

· 2 ·

Medication-Assisted Treatment (MAT)

What You Need to Know

The practice of trying to help individuals who are addicted to one substance by substituting another, less dangerous one, or by using medications in an effort to reduce cravings, has a substantial history. Today this practice goes by the name "medication-assisted treatment" or MAT. It is defined by the U.S. Food & Drug Administration as follows: "Medication-assisted treatment (MAT) is the use of medications in combination with counseling and behavioral therapies, which is effective in the treatment of opioid-use disorders (OUD) and can help some people to sustain recovery."[1]

Of note in the above definition is the phrase "in combination with counseling and behavioral therapies." In other words, if MAT is to be part of a newly sober person's recovery program, it should be done not in isolation but in combination with counseling and therapy aimed at making behavioral changes.

THE ARRAY OF TREATMENT OPTIONS

Treatment for addiction (or to use current terminology, a "severe substance-use disorder") was long associated with a 28-day stay in a rehab facility. But this has changed. Residential treatment remains the most expensive option, with some facilities charging $20,000 or more for a 30-day stay.[2] Intensive outpatient treatment, which requires the patient to attend treatment for several hours a day for several weeks, typically costs between $3,000 and $10,000 for 30 days. In contrast, MAT is

7

much less expensive, with methadone maintenance costing roughly $6,500 per *year* and buprenorphine treatment costing about $5,900 per *year*. These latter costs, which include brief case-management visits and drug testing, obviously cost much less than the more intensive forms of treatment, which is why family members can expect insurers to prefer and advocate for MAT.

Today it is highly likely that a man or woman in treatment for a substance-use disorder will find that medication of one sort or another is recommended as part of treatment and aftercare. This is especially true if the problem is opioid dependence, but it is also common for alcohol abuse. These medications, which we'll review shortly, can help a great deal, but again researchers have cautioned that they should not be relied upon as a total treatment package. Here is one such admonition: "Pharmacological interventions for opioid addiction are highly effective; however, given the complex biological, psychological, and social aspects of the disease, they must be accompanied by appropriate psychosocial treatments."[3]

For the newly sober person and his or her loved ones, the importance of the above statement cannot be overemphasized. Those who are reading this book must clearly understand and concur with the idea that because addiction is a complex disorder with biological, psychological, and social roots, so must recovery include all of these factors if the voyage that begins with rehab or treatment is to succeed. The ship that must cross those open waters successfully could be thought of as a three-masted schooner, as in figure 2.1. The biological, psychological, and social aspects of recovery would be represented by the three main sails. A fourth factor—the subject of this chapter—is MAT and could be represented by the triangular jib sails at the front of the vessel. Alternatively, you may wish to associate MAT with one of the larger sails. Regardless, it goes without saying, as sailors know very well, that a safe crossing of open waters requires all of these sails, working together. Trying to do it with one or more missing would be to invite disaster. Later we will dive more deeply into the issue of exactly what constitutes "appropriate psychosocial treatments." Suffice it for now to say that this condition is not satisfied by weekly check-in groups with a case manager who has no real therapeutic role.

It is well worth having a discussion between the newly sober individual and his or her loved ones about this idea of needing more than jib

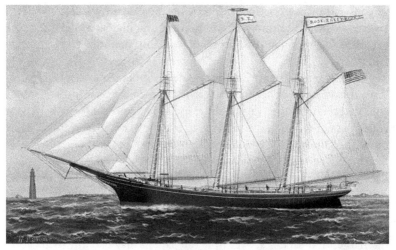

Figure 2.1. The Journey to Recovery. *Source: William Stubbs, 1842–1909. Public Domain.*

sails (i.e., medication) if MAT is to be part of a comprehensive recovery plan and if recovery is to be a safe crossing.

Let's now examine the most common forms of MAT in use today. You need to know how they work as well as what to expect (and not expect) from them.

Medications for Alcohol Abuse

The most common medication used to help individuals with alcohol-use disorders stay sober are naltrexone and acamprosate.[4] Naltrexone can be taken in two forms: a tablet that is taken daily orally or a monthly injection under the brand name Vivitrol, which is much more expensive than oral naltrexone. Naltrexone and acamprosate (available under the brand name Campral) are also sometimes used in the treatment of opioid dependence. With respect to alcohol, they work by blocking the euphoric effects associated with intoxication. Accordingly, they reduce cravings to drink. Research has found that taking either naltrexone or acamprosate can help individuals stay sober. However—and this is important—researchers also reported that compliance rates for both medications were low. In other words, many of those who are prescribed naltrexone or acamprosate do not take it daily or consistently as prescribed, thereby limiting the drugs' effectiveness.[5] In one study, for example, after one year roughly 60 percent of those prescribed naltrexone and 80 percent of those prescribed acamprosate had relapsed.[6]

Clinicians frequently report that newly sober patients who are prescribed naltrexone or acamprosate take the medication as prescribed for a limited time and then take it either inconsistently or not at all. This, of course, is not unique to naltrexone or acamprosate; rather, it is a common phenomenon associated with all sorts of medications prescribed for chronic conditions such as asthma and hypertension. And we must define alcohol dependence as a chronic condition. Just as a patient who is prescribed medication for hypertension may not meet with their prescriber very often, so the individual who is prescribed naltrexone as part of a treatment discharge plan may not be followed very closely after discharge. In both cases, over time the patient may take the medication either inconsistently or simply stop taking it.

Vivitrol is an injectable, long-lasting form of naltrexone that more recently has been approved for use in the treatment of opioid dependence. Like the oral form of naltrexone, it does not result in tolerance or withdrawal. However, as is also true for naltrexone, the injectable form does not result in feelings of euphoria as the drugs discussed below do. In an initial study it was reported that 90 percent of those patients who were treated using the injectable, long-lasting form of naltrexone remained abstinent from heroin.[7] So this is encouraging, though in this study patients were required to visit a clinic monthly in order to get their injection. This could have helped to increase medication compliance. Also, not all insurers today will pay for this form of naltrexone due to its significantly increased cost. Yet the fact that injectable naltrexone does not create a euphoric high may be a significant advantage.

So are we to infer that naltrexone is effective or ineffective? In reality, the best we can say is that these medications work if you take them. The issue, again, has to do with compliance (or what is called "medication adherence"). Obviously it is easier to stop taking oral naltrexone—either because a person becomes lazy about it or because they plan to use alcohol or opioids. This is not so for the long-lasting, injectable form. Again, the lesson to be learned here is what researchers studying opioid dependence advise: MAT should be accompanied by a more comprehensive recovery plan that can help, among other things, to increase medication compliance. This is precisely the theme of this book. This more comprehensive approach includes active collaboration between the newly sober person and his or her loved ones, who are equal stakeholders in recovery, along with ongoing treatment (preferably an evidence-based one).

Medications for Opioid Dependence

Methadone was the first medication created and marketed exclusively as a means of reducing the use of heroin. It has been in use since 1947 and therefore has the advantage of a large body of research that bears on its effectiveness. Methadone is an opioid, and people on methadone maintenance therapy do become addicted to it. It has the advantage, though, of not increasing the user's tolerance (such that he or she needs larger and larger doses to achieve the same effect) as does heroin. For many years, methadone clinics flourished in virtually every town and city in America. Typically, the man or woman on methadone would need to report to the clinic to get a week's supply (at most) of the medication. They might also meet briefly once a month with a case manager; however, it would not be accurate to qualify this contact as "therapy" or "counseling," as it did not address issues other than the patient's compliance with methadone—and whether a drug test showed them as positive for heroin.

So is methadone a good option for a newly sober man or woman following treatment or rehab for dependence on heroin or prescription opioids? This is a worthwhile discussion for the newly sober person and their loved ones to have, and there are a few facts that can inform such a discussion. First, studies show that methadone does reduce opioid (heroin) abuse. Specifically, patients taking methadone had approximately one-third fewer opioid-positive drug tests than a comparison sample of men and women not taking it.[8] While this is encouraging, it's also important to note that other researchers have found that roughly half of those on methadone test positive for opioid use as compared to a whopping 80 percent among those not taking methadone.[9] So the truth may lie somewhere in the middle. But the important thing to keep in mind is that if the newly sober individual, in consultation with loved ones, opts for methadone as a follow-up to treatment, he or she is clearly not out of the woods. As pointed out earlier, addiction is a complex problem. Biological, psychological, and social factors all contribute to it. This being so, it makes sense that a solid recovery plan would take all of these factors into account and address them. In contrast, relying solely on a medication, such as methadone, is no guarantee of a safe voyage into recovery.

Recently methadone has been increasingly supplanted by buprenorphine as a treatment for opioid dependence. Buprenorphine is prescribed either as is or in combination with another drug—naloxone—which is added because it prevents the individual from getting high if they attempt to misuse the buprenorphine, for example, by crushing the pill form of the medication. This latter combination drug goes under the name Suboxone. Suboxone is now also available in a sublingual form that melts quickly in the mouth. In either form this medication is in fact an opioid and therefore it has opioid-like effects on patients; however, like methadone, its effects are less than that produced by heroin, and patients don't build up a tolerance, which would result in needing to use more over time. Suboxone has an added benefit in that the patient does not need to report to a clinic to get a supply of it because it can be prescribed by virtually any licensed prescriber (including the patient's primary care provider).

So is Suboxone a miracle drug? That depends on whom you ask. Certainly for the newly sober individual who wishes to quit heroin or prescription opioid use, it offers a way out of that prison. But like methadone, Suboxone is not 100 percent effective. In one study, 60 percent of patients on the drug still tested positive for opioid use as compared to 90 percent who were not on the drug.[10] Another study was more encouraging, with roughly 25 percent of those taking Suboxone testing positive for opioid use.[11] And there is also a debate as to how long an individual should stay on Suboxone. Opinions vary, from those who advocate "Suboxone for life" on the one hand to those who regard Suboxone as more of a bridge to a healthier, substance-free lifestyle. In any case, Suboxone may be a good option to consider as part of an overall recovery plan for the newly sober person. That said, it would be playing with fire for either the newly sober individual or his or her loved ones to look solely to Suboxone as the answer.

REASONABLE EXPECTATIONS

What can those completing treatment, along with their loved ones, expect MAT to contribute to staying clean and sober? The answer is they can expect it to help as long as recovery is not based on MAT alone. Here is a typical case.

Jeanna's son, Mason, at age twenty-four had become addicted to heroin after starting, as many young people do, by abusing prescription painkillers. As a college student, Mason found these not very hard to come by. Unlike some others, however, Mason was never prescribed pain medication in response to an injury; rather, he got into them in the simple pursuit of pleasure. Before that he'd been a frequent cannabis user and occasionally had tried cocaine. But he found that the opioids gave him a high like no other. Mason believed that he had long suffered from what he called a low-grade depression stemming from his father's early death from a heart attack when Mason was thirteen. Nevertheless, he did well in school, graduated from college, secured an entry-level job, rented a studio apartment, and outwardly looked like he was well on his way to a successful life. But then the opioid use gradually caught up with him. Eventually he found that prescription opioids were too expensive so he used a friend to connect with someone who could supply him with heroin at much less cost. Of course, by then he was addicted. His performance at work slacked off so much that he was first counseled about it and then, six months later, let go. With no income, he had no choice but to move back with Jeanna, whom he told about his addiction and who called her doctor.

Mason was referred to an intensive outpatient program (IOP), where he spent several hours a day, four days a week, for six weeks. Mostly these were group therapy sessions where the primary subject was what the members were doing to stay clean. Some talked about going to AA or NA meetings; others talked about looking for work or staying busy at home. Weekly drug tests were used to check for heroin use. Part of the treatment was Suboxone, used as a substitute for the heroin. Mason was given one week's supply of Suboxone at a time, and he reported that he thought it was working. It did give him a little "high" he said—not a lot but enough to quell his craving for heroin.

After four weeks Mason was discharged from the IOP into a regular, weekly outpatient program operated by a local agency. His doctor now prescribed thirty-day supplies of Suboxone. He was also scheduled to meet with a case manager (not a therapist) every six weeks, at which time a drug test would take place.

At the second meeting with the case manager Mason tested positive for heroin. He was told that he could no longer participate in the regular outpatient group but would need to return at least briefly to the IOP.

This scenario is what, as a loved one of a newly sober individual, you might expect to face. For Jeanna this was immensely frustrating for several reasons. To begin with, she found it frustrating that she was told virtually nothing about what her son's IOP experience would entail. What did these groups focus on? What were the expectations for the participants, if any? Did her son suffer from any underlying psychological issues that should be addressed? She felt, she said, "totally shut out" when it came to what her son was going through to help his addiction.

Jeanna was also frustrated that she was told nothing about the medication that Mason was given or what to expect from it—this despite the fact that Mason had signed a document giving the clinic as well as the prescriber permission to communicate with her.

Finally, Jeanna was frustrated—and not a little angry—about not being included in decisions about what to do next for Mason despite the fact that he was living with her and did not seem to be doing anything constructive with his time.

The above scenario is totally antithetical to the theme of this book, which is that if recovery from addiction is to be robust it must address all of the factors that contribute to it and so is best approached as a *collaborative* effort between the newly sober person and his or her loved ones. In Mason's case this did not really happen. He was not able to name specific goals he was to work toward, specific lifestyle changes he would need to make in the interest of recovery, or even if he had made an honest decision about the need to pursue abstinence as opposed to "controlled use." In fact, his relapse was attributed precisely to his thinking that he could use heroin "safely, once or twice" as he put it. In effect, Mason was relying totally on MAT, while his mother was out of the picture.

As we move forward, this book will flesh out this collaborative approach with guidelines for how it can be accomplished. For now, the issue that the substance abuser needing treatment and his or her loved ones must confront is what kind of treatment seems appropriate. There are several factors to consider in this regard.

- What substances are we talking about? Alcohol? Heroin? Prescription opioids or other prescription medications? Cocaine? Methamphetamine?
- Is the substance user using one or more than one of the above?
- What kinds of consequences has the substance abuser experienced related to his or her substance use?
- Has the substance abuser been previously treated? If so, what form did this treatment take? Residential, IOP, MAT?

It can be disappointing when family members finally convince a substance-abusing loved one to enter treatment only to discover that the person approving their treatment appears to be recommending one that either does not seem to match the breadth and severity of the problem or is a repeat of a previously failed treatment. In this case it is very important that the concerned family members—who need to think of themselves as stakeholders in recovery—advocate for the level of care that makes the most sense to them. If cost is a factor, the family may need to consider whether they are in a financial position to subsidize a treatment an insurance company is unwilling to pay for. Finally, there is always an appeals process for addressing concerns.

It needs to be emphasized that the case of Mason points out how the recommended approach to treatment—specifically, to integrate MAT with a comprehensive treatment plan that includes appropriate ancillary treatments—seems to have been lacking here, as it often is. When this happens, the newly sober person and his or her loved ones need to come together to advocate for this kind of treatment. In Mason's case, for example, he could not recall ever being asked while in treatment to talk more about the low-grade depression he believed that he had long suffered from and whether it could be a risk factor for relapse if not addressed—either within treatment or as part of an aftercare plan.

Homecoming

Where the Rubber Meets the Road

*W*hether it is discharge from residential treatment or from an IOP treatment program, at some point the newly sober individual can be said to graduate from treatment—hence the title of this chapter. If entering treatment can be thought of as the point of departure for the voyage across open water that is recovery, returning to life following treatment could be said to be "where the rubber meets the road" as this is where the real work of recovery begins that will determine the outcome of the voyage.

At this point it's safe to assume that the vast majority of these men and women will have completed a course of treatment that has been deemed a success. It's also true that the assumption of loved ones (as well as those who conducted the treatment) is that the newly sober person is committed to staying sober—in other words, to abstain from the use of alcohol or drugs. In many instances this is true—at least at the point of the homecoming. The newly sober may express a commitment to staying clean. Assuming that this is true, the logical next question to ask the newly sober should be: How are you planning on achieving this? In other words, assuming for the sake of this book that the goal is to stay alcohol- and drug-free for at the very least one year following treatment, what is the plan for successfully completing the voyage from the point of departure through that year? Again, a statement of intention, no matter how sincere, may not prove to be sufficient. As pointed out in the last chapter, there is a 40–60 percent chance that the newly sober person will not stay sober. Without questioning motivation, it would be foolish to ignore this risk or move forward without a plan.

And that plan will work best if it is *collaborative* one between the newly sober person and his or her loved ones.

The first step that needs to be taken after homecoming is an honest assessment of exactly what the newly sober person's goal is. While many loved ones may assume that abstinence is the goal (which hopefully is the goal of treatment as well), the reality is that the newly sober individual may privately feel differently. Why is that? Well, some may still harbor a desire to or a belief that they still can use alcohol or drugs safely. Some will be frank in admitting this, but others may keep their belief secret for fear of disapproval. I've heard newly sober individuals leaving treatment say things like

- "I need to quit the opioids for sure but a little cannabis can't hurt."
- "Cocaine has caused a lot of trouble for sure but I don't see why I can't have a cocktail or two after work or on the weekend."
- "I'm taking an antidepressant now so I know that I'll never get back to using that much cocaine again, but a little cocaine now and then really helps me."
- "I've learned my lesson. I believe I can moderate my use now."
- "I'm through with heroin but I still need medication for my pain."

It can be more than a little difficult for a loved one to hear a comment like one of the above. In fact, these comments can evoke reactions ranging from panic to rage in the loved ones of the newly sober individual. Here is an example, as Camille explains.

My siblings and I all knew that Mom had a drinking problem for many years. For a time she actually functioned fairly well as a mother, despite her drinking, but over time she started falling asleep on the couch earlier and earlier after dinner. At that point she was not able to keep her attention on us kids for very long. So as time went on, we kids more or less grew up without a close relationship with her. Fortunately my father didn't drink to excess, and although he worked long hours as an accountant, he was more accessible. Between him and us kids we kept the household going.

My mother is a nurse, and for many years she never called out sick as far as I can remember, but at one point she injured her back trying to lift a patient who had fallen. After the surgery she was out of work for a month and unfortunately ended up getting hooked on pain killers. The hospital modified her work assignments somewhat to accommodate her reduced strength. But the worst part was that between the pain killers and the drinking she became less and less functional. She started missing work and was able to do even less than before at home. Later I learned that she was getting pain killers off the street, and that freaked me out. We finally all got together and decided that we needed to do an intervention. She tried denying that her drinking and drug use was that bad, but we persisted, and she reluctantly agreed to go to rehab.

As hopeful as we all were when Mom agreed to go to rehab, I found it very frustrating. Some of us went for a weekend family program, where we pretty much learned what we already knew about addiction, but we were also told that Mom had to be responsible for her recovery. The message seemed clear: we were basically being told to stay out of it—to mind our own business. After all those years of having to work around Mom's drinking, and then her opioid use, that pretty much pissed me off. I for one felt that I was as invested in Mom getting sober as she should be. Then in one phone call she told me that she knew she had to quit the opioids but then added, "But I think I could have a glass of wine at night, just to relax." I blew up at her, and the call didn't end well. Later I felt bad. Still, I wanted to tell someone that I thought my mother was contemplating making a deal with the devil but I had no idea who I could tell that to. I ended up making a call anyway to a counselor who listened, then thanked me for sharing that information. But I never heard back from him or anyone else on the staff, and when Mom came home, I just knew that she was thinking she could drink again, and that more or less made me lose hope.

Camille's mother did not intend to offend her daughter. On the contrary, she was expressing a belief shared by many men and women who complete treatment. Privately (and in Camille's mother's case, publicly) they are not fully convinced that they need to abstain from all substance use if they are to remain sober. In a word, they are *ambivalent* about the need to stay completely sober. Therefore I advise loved ones to consider this possibility and to maintain an open dialogue with the newly sober person in their lives. The key questions, of course, are "How committed are you to abstinence?" and "Do you really believe you can safely use any substances at all?"

CONTROLLED USE AND MODERATION:
WHAT DO WE ACTUALLY KNOW?

Today there are outside influences that can undermine the goal of abstinence following treatment for a severe substance-use disorder (and the reality is that if you are reading this book, it is a severe substance-use disorder we are most likely talking about, not a mild one). You may have heard about some of these so-called nonabstinence approaches. They tend to promote themselves as an alternative to abstinence by appealing to the idea that abstinence is too difficult a goal to achieve. Needless to say, to the person who harbors some ambivalence about whether he or she has been truly addicted and therefore needs to abstain, the idea that they can safely use is bound to be appealing. Some practitioners go so far as to advertise this as a goal if you seek treatment with them.

Ambivalence—especially about the need to change—is a common human experience. How many of us have at one time or another been advised that we need to change our behavior in one area or another? Typically, the more comfortable we are with that behavior, and the more it has become ingrained in our lifestyle, the less enthusiastic we're apt to be about making that change. We might reject the suggestion outright. Or we may seek to compromise: a little less red meat, fewer desserts, a little time exercising, less time on the internet, and so forth. This reflects simple ambivalence fully embracing the need to make a significant change in our lives. So it is when it comes to using alcohol or drugs. The difference is that when the issue is addiction, the stakes involved in ambivalence are very high.

As a newly sober person (as well as the loved one of a newly sober person), it is important to look beyond advertising that tells you that you don't need to quit. The best way to do this is to educate yourself about what the actual research has to say that can inform you on these options. Let's look at some of this research and what it has found.

Moderation

Moderation Management, founded by Audrey Kishline,[1] is a program that advertises that it supports men and women who want to moderate their use as opposed to abstaining. MM, as it is called, offers guidelines that include tables for tracking alcohol consumption and data on how much alcohol will be in a person's bloodstream depending on their sex, weight, and how much they consume. MM has a website (www .moderation.org) that includes a directory of meetings and guidelines for what it calls "responsible drinking."

A program like MM can have considerable appeal to someone leaving treatment who is not truly convinced of the need to abstain from substance use, and some of these men and women will admit to this. They may even challenge loved ones on the need to pursue abstinence. So what do we actually know about moderation, and how can this objective information inform the dialogue between the newly sober and his or her loved ones in a collaborative approach to recovery?

Some answers can be found in research conducted by Dr. Keith Humphreys, professor of psychiatry and behavioral sciences at Stanford University Medical School.

Dr. Humphreys and his team of researchers undertook to compare self-identified members of MM with self-identified members of Alcoholics Anonymous (AA). They looked at demographics—who attends AA versus who attends MM—as well as the relative severity of the drinking problems in the two groups.[2]

What Humphreys found, first, was that the severity of the drinking problems among those who preferred MM was significantly *less severe* than that of AA members. In effect, men and women who were drawn to MM had self-selected based on the fact that they had experienced mild to moderate, as opposed to more severe, consequences related to drinking. Therefore the two programs—MM and AA—seem to appeal to two different groups of people. In your case, would you say that your loved one who just completed treatment had a mild, moderate, or severe substance-use problem?

Additionally, members of MM were more likely to be female, younger than thirty-five years old, and employed. Those demographics cast MM membership as a pretty stark contrast to AA membership, which is much more diverse with respect to sex, age, education, and employment status.[3]

These researchers also found that the MM group as a whole was high on every social and demographic factor that has been found to be associated with being able to reduce drinking: being more highly educated, having full-time jobs, having family support, and so forth. In effect, MM members had the advantage of a social network that did not support heavy drinking but rather would support their decision to moderate. Based on these factors, the MM members had the most favorable prognosis for succeeding at moderation. But keep in mind: as a group they were very different from those who choose AA and abstinence over moderation.

One interesting finding from the Humphreys study is that about 15 percent of MM members reported that they had experienced three or more of the following symptoms at least once in the six months before they started going to MM: tremors (shaking when not intoxicated), delirium tremens, blackouts while drinking, convulsions after drinking, craving for a drink on waking up in the morning, and problems with their family or job as a result of drinking. These of course are all symptoms of a severe drinking problem, not a mild or moderate one. Despite that, only 3 percent of this 15 percent decided to pursue abstinence as opposed to controlled drinking as their personal goal through MM. There is no way of knowing how many of these individuals went on to suffer more severe consequences or who eventually elected to pursue abstinence. We do know, however, from her memoir, that Audrey Kishline herself eventually concluded that abstinence was her best option. Sadly, she was not able to sustain abstinence and ended her life via suicide.

In summing up, Dr. Humphreys states that the vast majority of MM members (85 percent) have low-severity drinking problems and also enjoy lifestyles that are conducive to reducing their drinking in lieu of stopping. At the same time, the other 15 percent are worrisome, leading these researchers to conclude that it would be unrealistic to recommend MM to all individuals who are experiencing problems related to drinking. With that provision in mind, moderation may be an acceptable goal for younger people who have stable lifestyles, who have social networks that do not support drinking, and who have none of the signs of alcohol dependence cited above (blackouts, cravings, etc.). In that case, MM may be a useful source of support.

Controlled Use

Another alternative to abstinence—essentially moderation by another name—is embodied in the idea of controlled use. This too has been the subject of research.

The first study we look at was undertaken by researchers from the University of California, Los Angeles, and Yale.[4] The participants in this study were 1,226 men and women, all of whom had been diagnosed as alcohol dependent (in other words, with a severe alcohol-use disorder) and who were part of a larger study that utilized a combination of therapy plus medication to treat them.

These individuals (428 were women) were recruited from eleven U.S. cities. At the outset, each of them was asked to identify their goal in seeking treatment:

- controlled drinking: "I want to use alcohol in a controlled manner —to be in control of how often I use and how much I use."
- complete abstinence: "I want to quit using alcohol once and for all, to be totally abstinent, and never use alcohol again for the rest of my life."
- conditional abstinence: "I want to be totally abstinent from all alcohol use for a period of time, after which I will make a new decision about whether I will use alcohol again in any way."

The treatment phase of this study lasted sixteen weeks and consisted of up to twenty individual sessions. An attempt was made to incorporate aspects from three evidenced-based treatment approaches: cognitive-behavioral therapy, Twelve-Step facilitation, and motivational enhancement therapy. These treatment approaches have all been found to be effective through controlled research studies. The outcome of treatment was measured in two ways: percent days abstinent (PDA) and drinks per drinking day (DDD). In addition the researchers also looked at how long it might take someone to relapse to heavy drinking, measuring this as days to relapse (DTR).

This was a large, national study. Multisite studies like this one have the advantage that their results are much less likely to be influenced by a particular form of treatment that may be favored by researchers at one particular university or treatment center. One could say that in multisite studies, such biases tend to "come out in the wash" while more robust results emerge.

What does this study have to teach us about the role that a person's goal might play in their recovery? Here is what the authors write in their discussion of their findings: "It was hypothesized that patients whose drinking goals were oriented toward complete abstinence would have better treatment outcomes as measured by a greater percentage of days abstinent, longer period until relapse, and an overall better clinical outcome. These hypotheses were supported by the present study."

To be even more specific, those men and women who chose abstinence as their goal had the best outcome after treatment while those with the goal of controlled drinking had the worst drinking outcomes. Finally, those who selected conditional abstinence as defined above had outcomes in between the two other groups.

In effect, this study suggests that the goal that a person sets out to achieve (when he or she decides to seek treatment as well as during homecoming) makes a difference when it comes to success, particularly for those with a severe problem. This is the decision that every newly sober person must face at homecoming. This research showed that a decision to seek to abstain was clearly associated with the best long-term outcome as measured by drinking versus not drinking and staying sober longer. Deciding on a goal of controlled use did not work out well because those in this group had the poorest long-term outcome. Finally, deciding to abstain for some period of time and then re-evaluate one's goal (conditional abstinence) appeared to lead to some sort of middle-ground outcome. We could conjecture that the choice of conditional abstinence as a goal reflects ambivalence—an internal wavering or uncertainty about the need to quit, period. But clearly a decision that one can successfully control substance use after being treated for a severe disorder does not bode well for long-term success.

A second study was conducted by Dr. William Miller of the Center for Alcoholism, Substance Abuse, and Addiction at the University of New Mexico.[5] Dr. Miller was interested in studying the effectiveness of a treatment program whose goal would not be abstinence from alcohol but rather moderation in drinking. With that in mind he set out, in collaboration with Dr. Ricardo Munoz of the University of California, San Francisco, to create and evaluate a treatment for drinking problems that they labeled "behavioral self-control" (BSC). This treatment is manual-guided, is delivered by trained professionals, and consists of a series of modules:

- goal-setting: What will the client's goal be for how much he or she drinks?
- self-monitoring: keeping a log of how much the client drinks each day

- self-reinforcement: learning ways to reinforce yourself for meeting your drinking goals
- identifying high-risk situations: What should the client avoid?
- alternatives to drinking: exploring other ways besides drinking of dealing with stress—for example, with anxiety or anger

Dr. Miller and his colleagues studied a group whose drinking problems would be considered severe. These individuals were evaluated at three, five, seven, and eight years after completing their behavioral self-control training. Of the 140 individuals (45 percent of them women) who began the study, 94 could be followed while 16 refused to participate in the follow-ups. The authors note that the status of those who dropped out could not be known. This phenomenon of course is familiar to researchers. For example, we cannot know the fate of those men and women who stop going to AA, or who drop out of treatment, and it would be inappropriate to count them as failures.

Let's look at what happened to the 94 who could be evaluated eight years after they completed BSC. Here is what the group led by Dr. Miller reported:

- 23 reported abstaining altogether from alcohol by choice (24 percent)
- 14 reported that they were able to control their drinking without significant consequences (15 percent)
- 22 had improved but were still impaired as a consequence of drinking (23 percent)
- 35 still had significant drinking problems and were classified as "unremitted"—in other words, as bad they were at the outset (37 percent)

What can we say about this effort at controlled drinking? First, it appears that a small minority of people (15 percent) were in fact able to reduce their drinking to a point where it was not causing a significant disruption in their lives. Does that mean that BSC doesn't work? No, though it does suggest that the BSC program can work for roughly fifteen out of one hundred people. Are those the odds that a newly sober wishes to bet on? For the majority though (61 percent), a decision to try to moderate their drinking left them either still impaired or no better off eight years later. Meanwhile, almost a quarter eventually decided on abstinence as their goal.

A footnote at the end of this study is intriguing. The authors comment that in their interviews with the men and women who failed to improve through their participation in behavioral self-control training, that failure was still not enough to motivate them to change their drinking goals and in particular to set abstinence as a goal. If you recall, that was true as well for the MM members who reported symptoms of a severe alcohol-use disorder. Some people, it seems, will cling to the belief that they can control their substance use no matter what. They prefer to continue to struggle and stumble for a long time rather than change direction. The best that can be said for both BSC and MM is that they appear to work for some people but that by no means are they a viable alternative to abstinence for everyone with a drinking problem.

DECISION TIME

Now that those individuals who have completed a treatment program for a substance-use disorder have returned to their home base, it's time for them and their loved ones to have a heart-to-heart discussion of exactly what goal the newly sober man or woman intends to pursue. This is no time for avoidance—for saying "Let's talk about it later," since later may prove too late. To cut to the chase, the decision boils down to this: Does the newly sober man or woman want to roll the dice and bet on their ability to succeed at moderation or controlled use, or do they think it better to place their chips on abstinence as a goal? Is controlled use or moderation a viable goal, or is it just wishful thinking? As it turns out, the answer to these questions depends on what kinds of substances the newly sober person was using and how severe their use was. Figure 3.1 may be helpful as a guide to this discussion.

As the diagram shows, substance use cannot be simply divided into two categories, namely, infrequent, low-risk use or severe, addictive abuse. Rather, substance use exists on a spectrum ranging from infrequent use on one end to severe abuse at the other end. Low-risk use does not imply no risk. It simply means the likelihood of advancing across the spectrum is low as long as the individual's use remains in that zone. So some people are able to enjoy a cocktail or two on a weekend

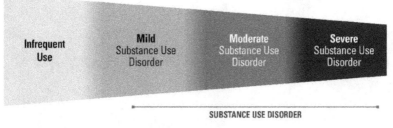

Figure 3.1. Substance-Use Spectrum. *Source: Author provided.*

or a glass of wine at night. In the same vein, it may be possible for a person to use cannabis on occasion. Alcohol, of course, is a legal substance while cannabis appears to be well on its way to being legal as well.

But does this mean that alcohol and cannabis are benign? Of course not. We are all familiar with the reality of alcoholism, and despite the popular notion that cannabis is harmless, cannabis addiction (or cannabis abuse disorder) is real.[6] In between infrequent (or low-risk) use and severe use are gradations of use. Typically, people who drink or use cannabis do not move quickly through these various stages. On the contrary, they more or less slip gradually from one stage to the next. Often they fail to connect the dots between their use and its accrued consequences on their health, emotional stability, relationships, family life, work performance, and so on. More often it's only when substance use has progressed to the moderate or severe level that consequences begin to become apparent.

For the sake of this discussion, it is probably best to assume that any substance-use disorder is in fact severe. This is usually the case for someone who enters treatment for an alcohol-use disorder, and it is almost certainly the case for those who have become ensnared in opioid or cocaine abuse. Still it can be useful for the newly sober and his or her loved ones to engage in a discussion of exactly where on this substance-use spectrum the substance user falls. Moreover, the discussion should include consideration of whether it is really safe for the substance abuser to consider controlled use or moderation of some substances given his or her experience with addiction. To be frank, the position taken here is that for at least the first year following treatment, abstinence from all substance use maximizes the chances of making a safe voyage into recovery for those whose use falls into the moderate or severe zones. To choose otherwise is to play with fire.

• 4 •

Preparing to Move Forward

Rethinking Enabling and Codependence

Enabling:

> In psychotherapy and mental health, enabling has a positive sense of empowering individuals, or a negative sense of encouraging dysfunctional behavior . . . In a negative sense, "enabling" can describe dysfunctional behavior approaches that are intended to help resolve a specific problem but in fact may perpetuate or exacerbate the problem. A common theme of enabling in this latter sense is that third parties take responsibility or blame, or make accommodations for a person's harmful conduct (often with the best of intentions, or from fear or insecurity which inhibits action). The practical effect is that the person himself or herself does not have to do so, and is shielded from awareness of the harm it may do, and the need or pressure to change.[1]

Codependency:

> Codependency is a behavioral condition in a relationship where one person enables another person's addiction, poor mental health, immaturity, irresponsibility, or under-achievement. Among the core characteristics of codependency is an excessive reliance on other people for approval and a sense of identity.[2]

> Codependency is a type of dysfunctional helping relationship where one person supports or enables another person's drug addiction, alcoholism, gambling addiction, poor mental health, immaturity, irresponsibility, or under-achievement, in order to satisfy the codependent's own emotional needs.[3]

29

The above definitions are the theme of this chapter. Both have come to have a common place in the parlance of addiction and, in particular, of the relationship between a substance user and his or her loved ones. As you can see, neither term is particularly flattering of these loved ones. On the contrary, they have come over time to have very pejorative connotations. For example, has anyone ever accused you or being an enabler? Has anyone suggested you suffer from codependency?

As negative as they are, these terms are common within the addiction treatment field. Examined closer, it's as though these terms actually place the responsibility for a substance-abuse problem on the loved ones rather than the substance abuser. They imply that loved ones actually make a problem worse.

Thankfully, despite their ubiquity, neither of these terms represents an official mental health diagnosis. You won't find them in the official publication that defines mental illnesses, *Diagnostic and Statistical Manual of Mental Disorders, 5th Edition* (DSM-5).[4] In other words, these pejorative terms may be mainstream in much of the writings on addiction, but they are not recognized as bona fide mental illnesses by the professional community. That's the first thing that the loved ones of newly sober individuals who are reading this book need to understand. You are not, in other words, responsible for your loved one's addiction or substance-use disorder. On the contrary, you are, much as is the addict, a victim of the disorder.

THE ORIGINS OF ENABLING

In order to get our heads around this idea of enabling, it can be helpful to get a sense of just how many loved ones of substance abusers there are out there. Based on the number of children with parents meeting the DSM-5 criteria for alcohol abuse or alcohol dependence, in 1996 there were an estimated 26.8 million children of alcoholics (COAs) in the United States, of which 11 million were under the age of 18.[5] As of 1988, it was estimated that 76 million Americans, about 43 percent of the U.S. adult population, had been exposed to alcoholism or problem-drinking in the family, either having grown up with an alcoholic, having an alcoholic blood relative, or marrying an alcoholic.[6] While growing up, nearly one in five adult Americans (18 percent) lived with an alcoholic. In 1992, it was estimated that one in eight adult American drinkers was an alcoholic or experienced problems as a consequence of his or her alcohol use.[7]

The above numbers are pretty staggering. But do they suggest that this many children and partners of individuals who have fallen victim to alcohol abuse are somehow responsible for it by virtue of having enabled it? The position taken here is clear: No, they are not responsible. In fact, it's only by disabusing themselves of any notion of having caused the problem that the loved ones of the newly sober can shed themselves of guilt and comfortably put themselves in the position of being equal stakeholders in the recovery process.

In its commonly used form, the concept of enabling refers to ways in which loved ones of substance abusers often unwittingly allow a substance-abuse problem to continue and even worsen. I say "unwittingly" because allowing the problem to continue or worsen is not the intention behind enabling. To illustrate this, consider the following examples of behavior that could be defined as enabling:

- Simply avoiding talking about a substance abuser's alcohol or drug use. In other words, promoting a conspiracy of silence around the problem. As one woman described it, "We all knew that Dad had a drinking problem. He was a reasonably successful attorney. He worked long hours. We weren't rich, but we didn't lack for anything either. Dad would come home from his practice, usually eat some leftovers from the fridge, and then sit in his recliner in front of the television. A table next to the recliner held his bottle of bourbon and a glass. Sometimes he'd get up to put some ice in the glass, but usually he just drank it straight. He was what I would call a 'sipper' in that he'd sip on his bourbon until he fell asleep. Then Mom would wake him up, and he'd go to bed. I can never recall any of us talking about Dad's drinking, much less confronting him about it."
- Making excuses for some of the consequences of substance use. For example, making an excuse for a spouse who is too drunk to meet friends for dinner or attend a social event.
- Providing money or purchasing alcohol or drugs for a substance user rather than taking the chance of allowing them to travel

to get it. "I recall my mother asking my older brother, who was then eighteen, to 'do her a favor' and go buy a six pack of beer for her when she'd run low."

- Assuming responsibilities that the substance abuser is unable to handle due to substance use. One young man explained, "My father was a daily pot smoker. He was a high school teacher and when he'd get home every day after work the first thing he'd do was to light up. And on the weekends he'd start up even earlier. He'd go into the basement to do this—I think maybe because he thought we wouldn't know. But of course you could smell the pot throughout the house. One result of this was that he really didn't do much around the house. I remember having to mow the lawn every weekend because we all knew he'd probably never get around to it."

The above are some typical examples of enabling, and they point to two themes. First, the loved ones of the substance abuser did not intend to make the substance-abuse problem worse, though they may have unintentionally allowed it to continue. Second, they avoided confronting the substance-abuse problem directly. This raises the question of why loved ones find themselves entangled in enabling.

Shame and Fear

If enabling is so harmful to the substance abuser in the long run, then why do so many loved ones end up caught in a web of enabling? If there are two words that capture the primary motivation for enabling, those words are "shame" and "fear."

Substance abuse and addiction have long been a stigma in our society. Much of that stigma can be attributed to the pre-scientific belief that addiction is not the complex bio-psycho-social disorder we now believe it to be but rather a symptom of weak or deficient character. In other words, addicts were long regarded as individuals who lacked morality and willpower. They were regarded as weak, lazy, or both. Little wonder that families were reluctant to admit to having a member who had a drinking or drug problem.

Although the stigma associated with substance abuse and addiction has subsided some in response to greater publicity about addiction's true nature along with the fact that influential people have come forward to acknowledge it, it is by no means extinguished. Therefore many family members may be inclined, as in the example of the alcoholic attorney above, to avoid recognizing or talking about the problem. Lingering stigma, then, can be one reason why a substance-use disorder may be shrouded in a conspiracy of silence within a family.

A second factor that plays a prominent role in motivating enabling is fear. This fear typically takes one of two forms: fear of retaliation by the substance abuser or fear of the possible consequences of not enabling. For example, a fifty-five-year-old man explained to his counselor that his twenty-five-year-old son was a severe alcoholic who could not keep a job and kept moving back home every time he was fired. He would then ask to borrow money, which his father knew would never be repaid. He was also divorced, with a young son, but he did not contribute to the boy's support because he usually spent whatever money he had on liquor. The counselor raised the issue of whether the father should consider not allowing his son to move back home, denying him money, or possibly both, the idea being that this might motivate the son to seek treatment for his alcohol abuse. The father responded that he'd had another son, seven years older, who had died at an early age of cirrhosis of the liver. Despite the obvious risks involved in continuing to support his surviving son, the father flatly told the counselor, "I don't want to lose another son, and I'm afraid of what would happen if I were to kick him out." In this case, the fear of the potential consequences of not enabling placed the loved one in a difficult bind.

In another case, a wife explained that her family was financially dependent on the salary her husband brought in through his job as a construction foreman. His job often required him to travel from home to a construction site. The problem was that at least once a month her husband would wake up hungover and could not get out of the house on time. Neither did he want to take the risk of making a call and sounding hungover. So he would pressure his wife to make the call and either explain that he had woken up with a migraine (a condition he did not have) and was running late or bedridden or that he had to take one of their children to a doctor's appointment and would be late getting to the site. Here again is an example of how the fear of potential consequences (losing a job) can motivate enabling.

The other fear factor has to do with fear of reprisal from the substance abuser. Take for example a woman living with a man who abused cocaine and would occasionally ask her for money for cocaine when he'd run out. This woman was on medical disability. Her boyfriend held the lease on their apartment, and she could not really afford to live on her own. The problem was that if she argued with her boyfriend about giving him money for cocaine, he'd respond by threatening to kick her out of the apartment. Under these circumstances she saw no option other than to give him some of her disability money.

Another common fear of reprisal is simply the anger that a substance abuser can express if denied access to their substance of choice. A spouse or partner might fly into a rage if questioned about their substance use or denied access to alcohol or drugs. Few people relish confrontations like this so this scare tactic often will work, and the intimidated loved one will back off or give in.

Viewed from the outside (and lacking an understanding of the underlying dynamics), it is easy to see why a so-called enabler might be seen as actually causing a substance-abuse problem by providing the means, excuses, or simple silence that allow it to fester. Indeed, many individuals report that they have been labeled enablers with this very connotation attached. "I've been told I'm an enabler," they often tell a counselor, as if confessing to some character flaw or worse—as if they were the villain in a substance abuse scenario. Being regarded as enablers may also explain why so many loved ones of substance abusers feel that they have been told to stay out of the treatment process. "Let us deal with the substance abuse" is the message they get either directly or implicitly, "just take care of yourself." As one husband expressed it, "I got the distinct impression from the staff at the rehab where my son was being treated that I was part of the problem and not part of the solution."

The approach taken in this book is just the opposite, and it begins by asking the newly sober individual to own up to the role they have played in creating their enablers.

The Grooming of Enablers

Family members and friends of men and women who develop a substance abuse disorder do not wake up one morning and decide that they want to facilitate that disorder by acting in ways that allow it to continue or worsen. Substance-abuse disorders do not appear instantly; rather, they tend to move along the substance-use spectrum we saw in chapter 3. For some substances, like alcohol and cannabis, the progression is generally slower, sometimes taking years to progress to the point where significant negative consequences (harm to health, job performance, family life, etc.) accrue to the user. For other substances such as opioids, cocaine, and methamphetamine, the progression can occur rapidly. In any case, a pattern of enabling by loved ones can emerge—but not because they wish the substance abuse to progress. Instead, it is the substance abuser who systematically and intentionally creates his or her enabling network by *grooming* his or her enablers. In other words, the substance abuser has a role to play in all of the behaviors described above under the heading of enabling.

If the voyage toward recovery is to be successful, the enablers in the newly sober person's life need to acknowledge those behaviors that constitute enabling, but the newly sober person must also acknowledge the role that he or she played in promoting that enabling. The truth is that substance abusers groom their enablers, and if they are to succeed in achieving a robust recovery, they need to own up to that and then resist any urge to repeat the pattern of grooming. Here are some examples of how a substance abuser can groom an enabler.

Guilt. This form of grooming most commonly consists of trying to lay blame for the substance abuse on a loved one with the goal of getting the loved one to enable the abuser's substance abuse. Readers who might identify themselves as enablers may relate to being accused of somehow having caused the problem. "I drink because my marriage is unsatisfying" or "I drink because our kids are out of control and it drives me crazy" or "I drink because it's the only way I have to wind down after having to work as hard as I do to support us" or "If you treated me better I might not have to get high every day." One woman described the way she was groomed to be an enabler this way:

> My thirty-year-old daughter has a severe problem with drinking and tranquilizers. But she blames me for this because I divorced her father—who was also an alcoholic—when she was ten. She claims that this was "traumatic" and the reason she needs to drink and take anti-anxiety medication, which she also clearly abuses.

Finally, a variation of this strategy of grooming utilizes guilt in the sense of making an enabler feel obligated because of commitment. "You took a marriage vow to be together for better or worse. So what if I drink too much? That's just who I am, and you need to accept that." Faced with such accusations, it is not difficult to see how loved ones may more or less back off rather than confront the substance-abuse problem for what it is. That in turn allows the substance-abuse problem to continue and worsen.

Fear.   Raising the specter of dire consequences is another way that substance abusers groom their enablers. "If you don't call in sick for me today, I might get fired and then where would our family be?" or "If you kick me out of the house, I won't be responsible for what happens to me." One man in his mid-thirties who already had a long history of alcohol and cannabis abuse, combined with a poor work history and financial irresponsibility, responded to his parents when they said they could no longer afford to keep him in an apartment, "If you can't help me pay my rent I have no place to go. I'll end up one of those people who live under an overpass." Or consider the successful attorney with a history of back pain who ended up hooked on prescription painkillers that his wife and two grown daughters knew he was buying off the street because his doctor would no longer prescribe them and had recommended a pain clinic instead. When they tried to confront him and get him to seek treatment, he replied that the pills were the only way he could get through the day and that he might have to leave the practice if he had to do without them. And as a final example, "We have to pay for a lawyer to get me off this DUI charge because if it goes on the record I'll most likely get fired."

Anger.   Simple anger can be an effective way of scaring enablers and getting them to not only avoid talking about their concerns about substance use but actually give in to the substance abuse. The substance abuser may fly into a rage at the mere mention of whether she or he is drinking too much or using too much pain medication. Physical violence is also not unheard of. Faced with such rage, many loved ones would sooner avoid the conflict and remain quiet—or even engage in some other means of enabling.

Drawing False Comparisons.   Another common strategy used by substance abusers to groom their enablers is to draw false comparisons between their own use and that of others. They might point to a friend who drinks more heavily than they do in an effort to downplay their own use. Another popular form of this strategy is to attempt to normalize the problem: "All of our friends like to drink, and most of them smoke pot as well." They might point out that someone they know abuses another substance or has had a problem with prescription opioids. The common message here to the enabler is "You're making too much of this. So back off."

Promoting Substance Abuse. "For a long time my partner tried to draw me into becoming his drinking and using partner. And for a time, I did fall into this. But then I started to see how this was just a cover for his own use. When I started to back away, the conflict between us over his use got steadily worse." This is a typical example of how a substance abuser can seek to groom a significant other by making them a drinking or using buddy.

GETTING HONEST

Recovery from substance abuse begins with getting honest. Previously we looked at how the newly sober man or woman needs to look inward and honestly assess the extent of his or her substance-abuse problem. They then need to get honest about what the best goal to pursue is: abstinence, or some form of moderation or controlled use.

The subject of this chapter moves us further in this process of getting honest, for the so-called enabler and the substance abuser alike. Enabling does not simply spring from the mind of the enabler. It can indeed promote the substance-abuse problem—usually unwittingly. But the substance abuser must acknowledge the role that he or she plays in grooming one or more enablers. Table 4.1, "Enabling Inventory," can be a useful tool for doing this.

The best way to approach using this table is as a way of beginning a conversation between the newly sober man or woman and a loved one who believes that they may have played a role in enabling the substance-abuse problem to continue or even worsen. Typically, enabling has this effect, however unintentionally. Yet it is important for the newly sober person's recovery that both enabling and the motivation or motivations behind it be recognized, in large part so that this can be avoided moving forward.

Table 4.1.   Enabling Inventory

Enabling Behavior by Loved One	What Motivated the Enabling?	How Did the Substance Abuser Encourage (Groom) the Enabling?	How Could the Loved One React Differently in the Future?

The other half of the "Enabling Inventory" addresses the newly sober individual and asks them to recognize and own up to the role they played in facilitating enabling. Which of the strategies described above did the substance abuser use in an effort to groom his or her enablers? This honesty is called for if the relationship between the substance abuser and his or her enabler is to change so as to promote recovery as opposed to relapse. Such a discussion may not be easy, but it's pretty obvious how important it is. The net outcome should be a sense of how the one-time enabler can and should behave differently in the interest of recovery.

CODEPENDENCE

The second popular concept that looms over recovery is that of codependence. Many loved ones of newly sober individual can attest to having been essentially accused of being codependent, virtually implying (as the definition cited at the beginning of this chapter suggests) that they somehow intentionally created and maintained their loved one's substance-abuse problem. Let's return to our definition of codepen-

dency above: "Codependency is a type of dysfunctional helping relationship where one person supports or enables another person's drug
addiction, alcoholism, gambling addiction, poor mental health, im-
maturity, irresponsibility or under-achievement, in order to satisfy the
codependent's own emotional needs."[8]

This view of codependency clearly implies that codependence is a
mental disorder and is a diagnosis in and of itself on the same level that
a substance-abuse disorder is an accepted psychiatric diagnosis. But to
be clear, this is not so. As one psychologist who conducted a rigorous
review of writings on codependence concluded, there is no consensus
definition of this term among professionals nor is there any solid body
of rigorous research that supports it.[9]

Another team of researchers took on the task of reviewing the
various definitions of codependence that exist in the literature. They
found that codependent individuals were most often described as self-
sacrificing and motivated to control other people with a tendency to
suppress their own emotions. The researchers concluded that although
these characteristics are commonly attributed to people considered codependent, "this does not provide evidence that an actual disorder exists."[10]

Finally, researchers studying a sample of college students who
identified themselves as codependent based on a preliminary checklist
were administered a series of tests aimed at identifying common characteristics. The only common trait the researchers were able to identify
was low self-confidence. They concluded that it was not possible to
predict very much about how such individuals might behave based on
this one quality alone.[11]

This finding regarding low self-confidence, combined with the finding of being self-sacrificing and tending to suppress one's emotions, does
not constitute a psychiatric diagnosis in large part because not all subjects
in these studies shared all of these traits and also because these characteristics might exist in many of us to one degree or another. However,
while they do not define an independent diagnosis, they may provide us
with a window of insight into why some people may be more vulnerable
to enabling than others. It's quite reasonable, for example, to imagine
how an individual lacking in self-confidence might be an easy target for
grooming as an enabler. The same would be true for an individual who
hesitates to express their feelings. Both the low-self-confidence individual as well as the individual who suppresses their true feelings would

be hesitant to confront a substance abuser and would perhaps fall victim to one or more of the grooming strategies we've reviewed.

What about the issue of codependents wanting to control others? That image does not comport well with having low self-confidence and a tendency to suppress one's true feelings. An alternate way of looking at this—and one that would seem compatible with what an enabler seeks to do—would be to posit that people who have been labeled codependent may simply be engaging in a kind of damage control that could be construed as controlling. For example, a wife who worries about and keeps tabs on her alcoholic husband and who insists on knowing where he is when he goes out might be seen as controlling, although her true motive would be ensuring she'll be able to find her husband if she believes he is out somewhere and drunk. The same would be true of the parent of an adolescent with a known substance-abuse problem who similarly tries to keep track of their teen's whereabouts and who they are with and even tries to place restrictions in these areas. Such a parent might also be seen as controlling. However, such a tendency to control may in fact be better thought of as a desire to minimize the potential consequences of their child's substance abuse.

WHAT TO DO?

Readers who find themselves identifying to some degree with this idea of codependency can begin the process of moving beyond it by doing an honest self-assessment to determine, first, if one or more of these elements does describe them and, second, how this might that have made them vulnerable to being groomed as an enabler. Next, they might seek help, either through finding helpful books, for example, about building self-confidence or learning to "find their voice." They might also benefit from personal counseling. After all, these traits might well interfere with their ability to get as much out of life as they could, independent of how they affect their relationship with the substance abuser.

The material covered in this chapter can best be thought of as an effort to "clear the decks" of factors that can undermine the recovery journey. This is best approached as a joint endeavor—a collaborative effort—by the newly sober person and his or her loved ones, who are equal stakeholders in recovery.

· 5 ·

Post-rehab Fellowships and How They Help

$\mathcal{N}$ow that the newly sober person has left the treatment or rehab facility that marks the point of departure for recovery, the question becomes: What happens next? The position taken in this book is that a lot needs to happen next. Recovery, if it is to be robust and resilient, requires change, and that change needs to include both the newly sober person and his or her loved ones who are stakeholders in that recovery process. For some newly sober individuals, this idea may be less than appealing—especially if they are harboring the idea that they can safely use the substance again or somehow moderate their use after suffering a severe substance-abuse disorder.

RADICAL INDIVIDUALISM: A BARRIER TO RECOVERY

Some newly sober individuals may also prefer to embrace the idea that they can beat a substance-use disorder all on their own. They act as if they believe that all they needed was treatment and that now they don't need any more help. In other words, even if they choose to pursue abstinence, they believe that their own willpower will be sufficient to get them there. To be blunt, however, research suggests that this is a dangerous notion and one that is more likely to lead to relapse than recovery. We'll look at that research shortly. But first let's examine the roots of this idea that a person can solve any problem, or overcome any handicap, all by themselves. This has to do with the concept of individualism, which can be defined as follows: "Individualists promote the exercise of one's goals and desires and so value independence and

41

self-reliance and advocate that interests of the individual should achieve precedence over the state or a social group."[1]

Individualism has long and deep roots in American culture, which has valued individualism from the time of the American Revolution. The prestigious *Brown Political Review* puts it this way: "The United States has one of the most individualistic cultures in the world. Americans are more likely to prioritize themselves over a group and they value independence and autonomy."[2]

American heroes such as Thomas Jefferson and Theodore Roosevelt are admired in part because of their championship of the idea and value of individualism. It shouldn't be all that surprising, then, that an individual—given our cultural tradition—could believe that he or she can beat a substance-use disorder without reaching out to or depending on others. But is this really a good idea when it comes to addiction?

A problem can emerge when individualism as a value morphs into a variant where we come to believe that we are each an island unto ourselves with no need at all to depend on others. Not all cultures see things this way. In Amish culture, for example, no man builds his own barn; rather, the community comes together for a collective barn raising. Similar traditions hold in other cultures. As another analogy, consider, as we do in this book, comparing recovery to crossing open water, like an ocean. There are, to be sure, a few individuals who have attempted such crossings solo. However, solo crossings are difficult and infrequent. When it comes to recovery, it is better to attempt such a crossing with the help of others. This includes loved ones, but it also includes "recovery fellowships." Recovery fellowships exist for the sole purpose of supporting individuals who have reflected on their experiences using substances and decided that abstinence is the best goal for them to pursue —and that reaching out is the best way to achieve that goal.

RECOVERY FELLOWSHIPS: WHAT THE RESEARCH HAS TO SAY

The most ubiquitous (but not the only) fellowship that exists to support abstinence and recovery is Alcoholics Anonymous (AA). Largely because of its widespread availability, AA has been the predominant focus of research that seeks to see how much participation in a fellowship can support recovery. It's safe to assume, I believe, that the results of this research apply equally to the other recovery fellowships we will look at more closely later. The purpose of including this summary of some of the most important research on recovery fellowships is simple: It is important that both the newly sober individual and their loved ones have accurate, factual knowledge when making decisions about moving forward after treatment. Unfortunately, and for better or worse, we live in the age of the internet, which does not by and large check material that is posted there for accuracy. Many posts that criticize one approach to treatment or recovery are actually little more than advertisements for the writer's preferred approach and are not necessarily based on evidence. Others reflect an individual's bias against an approach to recovery, such as AA. People are entitled to their opinions, of course, but readers of this book will be wise to be skeptical of claims that are not supported by rigorous research. Often a simple Google search will reveal if any such research exists to support a claim made on the internet.

The first study we look at was conducted by researchers at Stanford University.[3] This study began by identifying a sample of 362 men and women who had experienced enough problems related to drinking that they were motivated to call an information and referral center in an effort to get help. A diagnosis was then made on the basis of what they said about themselves and their drinking via a questionnaire. The researchers then followed these volunteers for sixteen years—a remarkable length of time for any study—assessing them periodically.

This group of men and women was divided at the outset into three categories depending on what each individual chose to do about their drinking. In other words, no one was assigned to any of these groups; rather, the groups simply represented the different pathways that the participants voluntarily chose to take in the first year of the study. Here are the pathways:

- group 1: people who decided to start going to AA but not to seek professional treatment of any kind
- group 2: people who decided to start going to AA and seek professional treatment at the same time
- group 3: people who decided to seek professional treatment but did not start going to AA

When examined "at the starting gate"—when they first entered this long-term study—the three groups did not differ demographically or in terms of their drinking patterns. For example, it was not found that men and women with the worst drinking problems chose one path over the others. This is important because it means, in effect, that the three groups were initially comparable other than in the different pathways they chose.

All three groups were followed and then assessed after year one, year three, year eight, and finally again at year sixteen. This is indeed a long time to follow a sample of people and is a good example of what researchers call a longitudinal study. Naturalistic longitudinal studies like this one have the potential to tell us a lot about the consequences of the different pathways that individuals choose to pursue. In the case of this study, here is what they found:

- People in group 2, who opted for treatment and AA at the same time, participated in AA longer and more frequently. Moreover, people in this group were the most likely to stay sober throughout the course of the study.
- People who dropped out of AA at any point after starting it were more likely to start drinking again.
- The longer people remained active in AA, the more likely they were to stay sober at all four follow-ups.

The newly sober man or woman and his or her loved ones who are reading this should give some thought to these results. Clearly a decision to get involved and stay involved in a supportive fellowship such as AA (or any of the other recovery fellowships we will review later) boosts the prognosis for recovery significantly. The combination of treatment plus involvement in a fellowship supportive of abstinence is the most powerful option in terms of long-term recovery.

One additional finding of interest concerned those in group 3, who opted at the outset for treatment but decided against going to AA. Some of the men and women in this group later decided to try AA. However, for them the late decision to try AA did not seem to improve their chances of staying sober. One of the things we know about this group, though, is that they attended AA meetings less often than those in the other groups even after they decided to give AA a try. The authors of the study conjecture that the men and women in group 3 may have had negative or skeptical attitudes toward AA—for example, that it encourages dependency. Alternatively, they may not have believed (rightly or wrongly) that their alcohol-use disorder was severe enough to warrant attending AA. Either way, these late starters did not fare as well as their fellow participants who opted either for AA or AA plus treatment at the beginning.

Another important study worth looking at was conducted by researchers of the Alcohol Research Group and the University of California.[4] They recruited 349 men and women (35 percent were women) from ten public and private alcohol treatment programs. While these individuals' drinking problems were severe enough to qualify them for treatment, they did vary to some extent in severity. The individuals of this group—who had never had treatment for drinking problems before—were then assessed one year, three years, and five years after finishing treatment. At each point they were asked how often they'd had a drink in the previous thirty days. This is a measure of drinking behavior frequently used by researchers and especially when study participants are to be reassessed at several different points in time. And it makes sense. If an individual consistently reports, at several different points in time, that she or he has been clean and sober for the previous thirty days, that can be taken as an indication that this individual's recovery is going well. Accordingly, those who report no drinks in the prior thirty days are then classified as "abstinent" (at the time they are assessed), while those who report having consumed even a single drink in that time period are classified as "nonabstinent."

As with the previous study, the researchers were interested in seeing how much these men and women had used AA and how that in turn related to their recovery. They defined what they called different "AA careers" as follows:

- Low AA involvement. This group mainly attended AA during the first year after finishing treatment.
- Medium AA involvement. This group continued to attend AA meetings at an average rate of sixty meetings per year after completing treatment.

- High AA involvement. This group also continued to attend AA meetings after treatment but at a rate of two hundred meetings or more per year.
- Declining AA involvement. This group was like the high involvement group for the first year following treatment but by the fifth year they were attending on average only six meetings per year.

These groups make for some interesting comparisons as the researchers assessed their rates of abstinence for the preceding thirty days at each of the follow-up points: one, three, and five years following treatment. Again, this kind of research has a lot to say to us about how involvement in a supportive recovery fellowship (in this case AA) relates to staying clean and sober.

The results of the five-year follow-up assessments were striking.

- 43 percent of the low-involvement group were abstinent at the time of all three follow-up assessments (year one, year three, and year five).
- About two-thirds of those in the medium-involvement group were abstinent at the year one follow-up, and this increased to 79 percent at the year five follow-up.
- 86 percent of the high-involvement group were abstinent at the year one follow-up, but this leveled off at 79 percent by the time of the year five follow-up.
- 79 percent of the declining group were abstinent at the year one follow-up, but this declined to 60 percent at the year five follow-up.

The message here once again is clear and unmistakable: greater involvement in a supportive fellowship is associated with better long-term outcomes for men and women initially diagnosed as having a severe alcohol disorder. Declining involvement, meanwhile, is associated with declining abstinence. However, in this sample at least, the added gain of attending two hundred or more AA meetings a year versus sixty was not as substantial as was that of extending attendance at the medium-involvement level beyond the first year following treatment. We might conclude, then, that if a person wants to maximize his or her chances of staying clean and sober, their best bet is to remain continuously and steadily active in a fellowship that supports abstinence at a rate at or above sixty meetings a year.

Another result of this study was that when asked at year five, over half of those in the declining group said they still felt like they were a member of AA. In other words, they still identified with AA despite the fact that they were attending few meetings. It is plausible to conjecture, then, that these men and women had internalized much of what they had learned during the time when their involvement in AA was greater, including a greater commitment to abstinence. A majority of this group was still doing fairly well, albeit somewhat less well than their more active peers.

Although there is actually a large body of clinical research that bears on the role of supportive recovery fellowships, let us review just one more, again for the purpose of allowing the reader to make informed decisions about moving forward after rehab. The *Journal of Substance Abuse Treatment* in 2014 reported on the results of an ambitious nine-year study of how attendance at supportive fellowship meetings following treatment for an alcohol-use disorder was related to recovery.[5] This study is important to look at for a number of reasons, the first being its comprehensiveness. A total of 1,945 men and women who underwent outpatient or inpatient treatment were recruited for the study. This large group was then assessed one year, five years, seven years, and nine years following treatment. They reported on how frequently they attended fellowship meetings and how much and how often they drank. Their self-reported behaviors were further validated by random urine screens.

This study is important for a second reason in that it represented a collaborative effort between an academic institution and the Kaiser Permanente Health Care System, a large, nonprofit health care provider. The participants, significantly, were all men and women who had health insurance that covered their treatment. In effect, this was a sample of middle-class Americans who had decided they needed help with a drinking or drug problem.

This group of men and women found their way into treatment via different pathways: through medical providers at Kaiser Permanente, through employee assistance programs, and also through their own initiative. During treatment they were required to attend at least one recovery fellowship meeting a week, but after treatment was over, they were on their own. The fellowship groups included AA as well as

Narcotics Anonymous (NA), Cocaine Anonymous (CA), or any other fellowship that supported abstinence. Understandably, 12-Step fellowships were the most available.

Also unique to this study was the way the researchers were able to analyze the data they collected. Not to get too complex, they were essentially able to determine not only whether fellowship attendance over time was predictive of recovery but also whether the reverse might be true; in other words, they were able to determine whether it is fellowship involvement that promotes abstinence or whether it is being clean and sober that actually causes people to go to meetings. Here is what they found: "Our results showed that greater 12 step meeting attendance led to increases in 5-year abstinence and to a lesser extent in 7-year abstinence. Causal associations in the reverse direction were not detected for those years."

These results make it clear that it is not being sober that somehow makes a person get involved in AA or another fellowship that supports abstinence; rather, it is getting involved in a fellowship that accounts for recovery. The authors conclude with this comment: "Importantly our analysis extends findings to a diverse population of treatment seekers, namely men and women with alcohol- and drug-use disorders who were insured members of an integrated health care organization."

Rigorous scientific research on the role of fellowships such as AA in supporting recovery from substance abuse is substantial and unequivocal. Still, AA continues to be the object of criticism. These critiques primarily take the form of personal testimonials from men and women who write about bad experiences they had or why they feel that AA didn't help them. Indeed, these individuals may not have liked AA, but their experiences are not consistent with the evidence just reviewed. A recent comprehensive review of the entire body of research, which included Twelve-Step facilitation (TSF), an intervention designed to foster AA involvement, had this to say:

> In conclusion, clinically-delivered TSF interventions designed to increase AA participation usually lead to better outcomes over the subsequent months to years in terms of producing higher rates of continuous abstinence. This effect is achieved largely by fostering increased AA participation beyond the end of the TSF intervention. AA/TSF will probably produce substantial healthcare cost savings while simultaneously improving alcohol abstinence.[6]

The bottom-line conclusion we can reach from all of this research is this: Going it alone is not the best choice following rehab. Using this knowledge, the newly sober individual must make two critical decisions. The first critical decision, covered in chapter 3, is whether he or she wishes to bet on his or her ability to moderate or control the substance-abuse problem that landed them in treatment versus deciding to pursue abstinence as a goal. The second critical decision, covered here, is whether they want to bet their future on their ability to sustain recovery on their own, and without reaching out to others, versus reaching for the support of others to help them maintain their recovery. The facts seem clear, but the choice is up to the newly sober individual—and to the extent that they are stakeholders in recovery, to his or her loved ones.

RECOVERY FELLOWSHIPS: OPTIONS

Although research on the role of participation in a recovery fellowship has focused mainly on AA due to its widespread availability, there is no reason to believe that a decision to get involved in another fellowship that has the same goal—supporting abstinence from substance use—would not have comparable effects. Here we review three such fellowships, beginning with the ubiquitous AA.

Alcoholics Anonymous

AA is a decentralized fellowship that was started in 1935 by a stockbroker and a physician who both acknowledged that they had lost control of their drinking and who found that meeting together frequently and talking helped them to stay sober. Though AA has a central office, that office exerts minimal influence over the fellowship as a whole. Registering with the central office is optional, and many meetings choose not to. This decentralization has allowed AA to grow, adapt, and diversify to a remarkable extent.

A few important facts to know about AA include

- Leadership at meetings rotates among the group's members, often on a monthly basis. AA is guided by its 12 Steps and 12 Traditions as opposed to any central authority.[7]

- AA is sometimes mistaken for a religion, which it is not. AA by tradition is intentionally nondenominational. In fact, its founder, Bill Wilson, was a lifelong agnostic. That said, AA could be called a "spiritual" fellowship to the extent that its traditions and steps support spiritual values such as honesty, humility, and altruism.
- While AA was started by and for alcoholics, today it is relatively easy to find meetings where members are working to abstain from other substances as well as alcohol.
- Although the use of opioids (such as Suboxone) to treat addiction to opioids is controversial, AA recognizes that some members require medication of one kind or another and supports this with the provision that the medication is prescribed.[8]

A visit to the AA website (www.aa.org) will reveal a list of meetings that, depending mainly on the population in any given geographic area, might include meetings specifically for men, for women, for gay individuals, for professionals, and so on. Today there is even a "secular" AA organization (www.secularaa.org) that describes itself as follows:

> We are an International Organization that supports the Secular AA Community. Our mission is to assure suffering alcoholics that they can find sobriety in Alcoholics Anonymous without having to accept anyone else's beliefs or deny their own. Secular AA does not endorse or oppose any form of religion or belief system and operates in accordance with the Third Tradition of Alcoholics Anonymous.

There is also a variety of meeting types, such as "open meetings" that are—as the name suggests—open to anyone, including those who are uncertain about whether they are truly alcoholics. These meetings are also open to loved ones of alcoholics who want to gain some insight into what AA meetings are like. Conversely, "closed meetings" are for men and women who have taken Step 1 of the AA 12-Step program and admitted that they are indeed alcoholics. So-called step meetings typically focus on a discussion on one of the AA 12 Steps, with members sharing thoughts on how they are "working"—in other words, following—that step in their daily lives. "Speaker meetings," meanwhile, follow the format of a recovering member telling their story of addiction and recovery, including the consequences they suffered due to addiction, what motivated them to reach out for help, and what their life is like now.

AA by tradition does have some rules of the road. These include, of course, personal anonymity (first names only are used at meetings) as well as a prohibition on "cross-talk," such as interrupting a person who is speaking. Interestingly, this latter tradition is consistent with typical rules that are observed in Native American talking circles, through which families and even communities identify and address problems.[9]

Many AA members report that they initially shopped around for meetings until they found one or two that they felt most comfortable in. Eventually they settled on a home meeting that they committed to attending regularly. They then reached out for a sponsor, who is someone they have no romantic or sexual interest in, someone who has been clean and sober for some time and who will serve as a guide (though not a therapist) to learning more about the fellowship's traditions. The sponsor also serves as a contact person to support recovery.

AA does not conduct or fund research into its effectiveness in part because by tradition it sees itself as a program of attraction, as opposed to mandation, as well as a fellowship as opposed to a treatment program. However, AA has conducted voluntary surveys on an average of once every three years since 1977. A review of the 2014 membership survey[10] reveals the following:

- Worldwide, there are some 115,000 active AA groups, but this figure does not include groups that choose to not register with the AA central office.
- AA membership (which began as a fellowship established by and attended mainly by men) today consists of 62 percent men and 38 percent women.
- 63 percent of AA members are between the ages of 31 and 60.
- 27 percent of AA members report being sober between six and twenty years while 22 percent report being sober longer than that.
- 86 percent of members report that they have a home group that they are committed to and that on average they attend about 2.5 meetings per week.
- After starting AA, 58 percent of AA members report that they have pursued some form of concurrent counseling to help them stay sober.

- 82 percent of members report that they have an AA sponsor, and 74 percent state that they got that sponsor within ninety days of starting to attend AA.

This last item from the AA membership survey, on sponsorship, is worth a closer look. AA has long advocated that new members get a sponsor, and soon, but researchers at the Center for Alcoholism, Substance Abuse, and Addictions at the University of New Mexico wanted to see if it was possible to see just how much of a difference sponsorship might make in recovery.[11] Specifically, they wanted to know how important it might be to have a sponsor very early in recovery, as recommended by AA, as opposed to after a person has been attending AA meetings for some time. To do so they recruited a group of men and women who had just begun to attend AA and then followed that group. For this study, to be sure that their sample was limited to AA beginners as opposed to more long-time members, prospective participants were excluded if they met one of the following criteria:

- more than sixteen weeks total lifetime exposure to AA
- abstinence from alcohol for twelve months or more after deciding that their drinking was a problem

Using these criteria, the researchers were able to identify 253 eligible participants (62 percent male) who had alcohol-use disorders but who were only beginning to utilize AA. They then used a measure called the Alcoholics Anonymous involvement scale (AAI). The AAI is a measure not just of AA attendance but of AA involvement, including whether or not a person has a sponsor.

After being recruited into the study, these 253 men and women were followed for twelve months. They were asked to complete the AAI at three months, six months, nine months, and twelve months. In addition, the study assessed sobriety. The results thus enabled the researchers to look at how a behavior such as having a sponsor might relate to staying sober during this initial stage of recovery. Moreover, they could then compare how having a sponsor very early (months one to three) might compare to having waited to get a sponsor (for example, for four to six months) with respect to abstinence. Along the way they could also look once more at whether AA involvement in general predicted recovery. What they found was remarkable: Getting an AA sponsor early (within the first three months) increased the probability of complete abstinence at months four to six nearly threefold!

The above AA membership survey statistics have been pretty much consistent since AA started conducting its triennial surveys. Though they do not constitute research in the sense of the academic research studies we've reviewed, they are nevertheless pretty much in line with the results of these studies. Taken together, they also offer a set of target goals for the newly sober man or woman who wishes to include AA as their recovery fellowship of choice in their post-rehab recovery plan. Just as important as it is for the newly sober individual to embrace these goals if their voyage to recovery is to succeed, loved ones are well informed to keep them in mind as well.

SMART Recovery

SMART Recovery (www.smartrecovery.org) describes itself as follows:

> SMART Recovery is an abstinence-oriented, not-for-profit organization for individuals with addictive problems. Our self-empowering, free mutual support meetings focus on ideas and techniques to help you change your life from one that is self-destructive and unhappy to one that is constructive and satisfying. SMART Recovery does not use labels like "addict" or "alcoholic." We teach scientifically validated methods designed to empower you to change and to develop a more positive lifestyle.[12]

Although SMART Recovery states that it does not use terms like "alcoholic" and "addict," their use of the term "addictive problems," along with their stated goal of promoting abstinence, does not seem to differ materially from the goal of AA as given. SMART states that it seeks "to empower people to achieve independence from addiction."[13] It seeks to do so through what it calls a 4-Point Program[14] that includes the following elements:

1. Building and maintaining the motivation to change
2. Coping with urges to use

3. Managing thoughts, feelings, and behaviors in an effective way without addictive behaviors
4. Living a balanced, positive, and healthy life

Like the other recovery fellowships we are looking at, SMART Recovery relies heavily on group support to achieve its objectives. The website includes a search page (www.smartrecoverytest.org/local/) that allows the reader to locate meetings by entering his or her geographic location. The focus of SMART meetings is on one or more of the above four objectives and how members can be working to make progress on them in their daily lives. The fellowship is a nonprofit organization and again, like AA, relies on a tradition of passing the hat at the end of meetings to collect money for things such as rent for using space or to provide small amenities such as nonalcoholic beverages or snacks.

Unlike AA, SMART meetings are run by trained volunteers, some of whom may be in recovery and others who are not. SMART offers online training for this purpose[15] for which it charges $99 and that takes approximately thirty hours to complete. The training includes education in the SMART 4-Point Program and the purpose as well as the limits of the SMART facilitator's role and guidelines for running meetings.

Both AA and SMART offer links on their websites to online meetings. These can be helpful to individuals for whom transportation may be a barrier to participation as well as to those individuals who suffer from social anxiety and for whom participating in an actual group would be otherwise challenging.

SMART claims that its program is supported by research. Unfortunately, most of this research consists of follow-up questionnaires completed by SMART members. Such research, conducted and reported on by a program that has an obvious interest in the success of the research, is not generally considered rigorous scientific research. One review of research on SMART Recovery[16] came to the following conclusion.

> Twelve studies (including three evaluations of effectiveness) were identified. Alcohol-related outcomes were the primary focus. Standardized assessment of non-alcohol substance use was infrequent. Information about behavioral addiction was restricted to limited prevalence data. Functional outcomes were rarely reported. Feasibil-

ity was largely indexed by attendance. Economic analysis has not been undertaken. Little is known about the variables that may influence treatment outcome, but attendance represents a potential candidate. Assessment and reporting of mental health status was poor. Although positive effects were found, the modest sample and diversity of methods prevent us from making conclusive remarks about efficacy. Further research is needed to understand the clinical and public health utility of SMART as a viable recovery support option.

Despite the limitations cited in the above review, the methods and goals that SMART relies upon are ones that could be said to be part of mainstream psychological treatment. In addition, SMART is a fellowship that relies on group support to pursue abstinence from substance abuse. And while rigorous research on SMART may still be lacking, the fellowship's goals and methods would appear similar enough to those of AA (including the goal of leading a "balanced, positive, and healthy life") that the newly sober individual and his or her loved ones might legitimately consider it an alternative to AA should it appeal to them more.

Women for Sobriety

Women for Sobriety (WFS; www.womenforsobriety.org) was founded by Jean Kirkpatrick, a sociologist, in 1977. Like Bill Wilson, the founder of AA, Kirkpatrick was an alcoholic who suffered consequences including severe depression, arrests for drunk driving, and two suicide attempts.[17] She also abused prescription drugs and amphetamines. Also like Wilson, Fitzpatrick had an epiphany at the point when her situation was most dire—in her case, picking up and reading a book by Ralph Waldo Emerson.

As the name implies, WFS is a fellowship for women who seek abstinence from substance use.[18] Its overview states, "WFS believes that having a life-threatening problem with alcohol and/or drug abuse is not a moral weakness, it is the symptom of a serious disorder which demands rigorous attention to healing."

In this regard WFS mirrors the AA belief that recovery requires rigorously "working" its 12 Steps. And like both AA and SMART Recovery, WFS relies heavily on group support to help its members achieve the shared goal of abstinence. The AA, SMART, and WFS home pages each also include a link whereby readers can locate meetings in their geographic area.

While AA seeks to pursue abstinence based on its 12 Steps and Traditions, WFS is based on what it calls six Levels of Recovery and thirteen Acceptance Statements. The Levels of Recovery are as follows.

Level 1: Acceptance of having a Substance-Use Disorder, one that requires the cessation of substance use.
Level 2: Discarding negative thoughts, putting guilt behind, and practicing new ways of viewing and solving problems.
Level 3: Creating and practicing a new self-image.
Level 4: Using new attitudes to enforce new behavior patterns.
Level 5: Improving relationships as a result of our new feelings about self.
Level 6: Recognizing life's priorities: emotional and spiritual growth, self-responsibility.

The WFS Acceptance Statements are[19]

1. I have a life-threatening problem that once had me.
   I now take charge of my life and my well-being. I accept the responsibility.
2. Negative thoughts destroy only myself.
   My first conscious sober act is to reduce negativity in my life.
3. Happiness is a habit I am developing.
   Happiness is created, not waited for.
4. Problems bother me only to the degree I permit.
   I now better understand my problems. I do not permit problems to overwhelm me.
5. I am what I think.
   I am a capable, competent, caring, compassionate woman.
6. Life can be ordinary or it can be great.
   Greatness is mine by a conscious effort.
7. Love can change the course of my world.
   Caring is all-important.
8. The fundamental object of life is emotional and spiritual growth.
   Daily I put my life into a proper order, knowing which are the priorities.

9. The past is gone forever.
   No longer am I victimized by the past. I am a new woman.
10. All love given returns.
    I am learning to know that I am loved.
11. Enthusiasm is my daily exercise.
    I treasure the moments of my New Life.
12. I am a competent woman, and I have much to give life.
    This is what I am, and I shall know it always.
13. I am responsible for myself and for my actions.
    I am in charge of my mind, my thoughts, and my life.

WFS is a recovery fellowship in that it relies on face-to-face meetings of peers who typically meet weekly for mutual support. Some online meetings are also available and can be located through the WFS home page. WFS observes a rule of anonymity as does AA. WFS relies on "certified moderators" to lead meetings. These are women who have at least one year of sobriety, have completed an application demonstrating an understanding of the Levels of Recovery and Acceptance Statements, and have been approved by the WFS organization. As another nonprofit organization, WFS relies on passing the hat and modest donations to cover individual meeting expenses.

WFS meetings follow a prescribed format beginning with a reading of the Acceptance Statements. The meetings are then similar to AA discussion meetings in that the moderator selects an issue from WFS literature to discuss. Meetings then end with members joining together to share aloud the WFS motto "We are capable and competent, caring and compassionate, always willing to help another, bonded together in overcoming our addictions."

NO EXCUSES: THE CHOICE IS YOURS

WFS represents a third alternative fellowship that exists for the sole purpose of supporting individuals who elect to pursue abstinence. Of these three, AA and WFS in particular were founded by individuals who had personally experienced the devastation of addiction and gone on to create solutions to it. But these solutions depend on two things:

- an honest look inward and a decision that abstinence, as opposed to moderation or controlled use, is the best goal to pursue based on the individual's experience with substance use
- a willingness to be humble enough to accept that personal willpower usually has not proven sufficient to overcome the problem and that reaching out to peers is the better choice

At this point the newly sober man or woman reading this guide, along with his or her loved ones, has reached another crossroads. The first was whether to recognize the severity of their substance-abuse problem and the choices needed to move forward. The second, now, is whether to accept their need for support from others in pursuing abstinence. Common arguments against this include things like

- I'm too busy—This is the most transparent excuse for not taking advantage of a group that can help the newly sober individual stay sober.
- Meetings are inconvenient—As noted earlier, every recovery fellowship includes lists of meetings as well as internet access to these lists and often the meetings themselves. It stretches the imagination that a newly sober person cannot find a meeting that he or she can get to.
- I don't feel comfortable in groups—Social anxiety is a reality, but there are online meetings that can be a starting place for such individuals.
- I'm not like the others in this group—This reflects an attempt to draw contrasts between the newly sober individual and others in a supportive fellowship. The business executive, for example, may claim that he or she can't relate to the blue-collar people at a meeting. A college professor may make a similar claim. Or the newly sober person may assert that the others at a meeting are much worse than they are.

All of these strategies boil down to an attempt to resist identifying with others in a fellowship by focusing on perceived differences as opposed to the primary commonality: pursuing abstinence from substance abuse.

All of the above are also transparent excuses for not giving one or more support groups a try and sticking with it for a while or shopping around for one or more meetings the newly sober person feels comfortable in. The actor Alec Baldwin, in an interview about his personal recovery from substance abuse, described his experience: "God got me sober. That day, God was a black, 65-year-old retired postal worker named Lenny . . . Lenny said, 'You never have to feel this way again if you don't want to.'"[20]

Loved ones are wise to not accept excuses but rather hold the line when confronted with them. To accept one or more of them portends danger for the voyage to recovery.

· 6 ·

Creating a Recovery Lifestyle

Part 1: People

𝒥n the previous chapters we discussed the possible role of medication in facilitating early recovery as well as the issue of just how much the newly recovery man or woman is committed to quitting alcohol or drug use. Then we looked at the role that support groups such as AA, SMART Recovery, and Women for Sobriety can play in supporting the pursuit of abstinence. But that is not where the voyage to recovery ends. The truth is that as substance abuse progresses, it tends to distort the user's lifestyle. Specifically, as substance abuse progresses along the substance-use spectrum described earlier (see chapter 3), substance use tends to play a more and more central role in that lifestyle. Another way to look at substance use is in terms of a relationship. It is important to take an honest look at just what kind of relationship the substance user had with his or her substance of choice at the time he or she entered treatment or rehab.

RELATIONSHIPS WITH ALCOHOL OR DRUGS

You will recall that we discussed the substance-use spectrum, which goes from low-risk use at one extreme to a severe substance-use problem—or what used to be commonly referred to as addiction—at the other extreme. You may want to take a moment to look back at that diagram in chapter 3 (figure 3.1). In between the two extremes are gray areas that we can call mild and moderate substance-abuse problems. Also, recall that these areas are not separated by sharp lines. In other words, men and women don't simply jump from one stage of substance use to the next. Rather, they move along this spectrum over time. With some substances, like cocaine and heroin, this movement can occur rapidly, while with others, like alcohol or cannabis, the movement tends to be more gradual. In fact, in the latter cases the individual may not notice the movement—though their loved ones eventually do.

The three stages of substance use—or relationships—are "casual friendship," "a serious relationship," and "commitment." Let's talk about how these types of relationships describe the changes that the substance abuser is likely to go through and how loved ones are likely to react at each stage.

Casual Friendship

- drinks or uses almost always in social situations and only occasionally alone
- rarely, if ever, appears clearly drunk or high
- shows no significant personality changes when drinking or using versus not drinking or not using
- maintains a functional lifestyle (family, work, etc.)

At this casual friendship stage of substance use, loved ones and friends may be aware that the user likes to drink or smoke or even on occasion use prescription or nonprescription drugs for recreational purposes. This is common, for example, among college students. This level of use rarely affects the user's ability to function—for example, as a family member, on the job, or at school. Loved ones and friends are therefore most often inclined to take a tolerant attitude toward someone in a casual friendship with alcohol or drugs. If the relationship remains at this level, it is not likely to pose a major problem. However, because the lines separating the different stages of substance use, as well as the different types of relationships, are not sharply defined, the individual may slip over time into the next type of relationship.

A Serious Relationship

- drinks or uses alone as often as or more often than in social situations
- drinks or uses to feel good or drinks or uses to relieve stress or anxiety

- shows noticeable personality changes when using versus not using, changes such as becoming more outgoing, less shy, more assertive, lethargic, and irritable
- gravitates toward people, places, and activities where alcohol or drugs are fairly accessible
- drifts away from activities that were previously part of his or her lifestyle such as hobbies and exercise
- may have "unexplained" medical problems
- begins to show deterioration in overall functionality (work, school, home life)

When the relationship to substance use has become serious, the user likes to have his or her substance of choice available and may go to pains to see that it is. The drinker may take to buying cases instead of bottles of wine or liquor. The cannabis user will be sure to maintain his or her supply. The opioid user will become noticeably anxious if he or she is running low and may begin to make "drug runs" to secure a supply. Loved ones typically notice these changes because they will be affected by them as well. As one woman put it,

> Fred refuses to go to any parties where he can't smoke pot. Since some of our friends don't indulge, that means we haven't seen them for a while, though I still sometimes see a couple of the women. I felt I had to explain the situation to them, and they've been supportive.

A daughter described her elderly mother this way:

> Mom likes to eat out, but she makes sure we always go to a restaurant that has a bar, and she has several cocktails during dinner. By the time dessert comes, she's drunk. We don't invite others to dinner to avoid the embarrassment of them seeing her drunk.

Some significant others may begin to feel jealous as they recognize the user's relationship with alcohol or drugs, and they may resent it because it is affecting their life as well as that of the user. Occasional comments are not unusual at this point, and they can lead to arguments. And at this stage, substance use begins to interfere with other roles such as that of spouse, parent, or employee. Household responsibilities may be ignored, interaction between spouses or between parent and child may wither, performance reviews at work may decline along with increased absenteeism, and so on.

Another frequent consequence of substance use when it reaches the serious relationship stage is that medical issues may arise. This is particularly true for alcohol abuse. Hypertension, early signs of diabetes, and declining liver function may begin to show up on annual physicals. If the progression along the substance-use spectrum has been gradual, the substance user may fail to connect the dots between drinking and these medical consequences—but again, loved ones may do so and become alarmed. Here again, discussions along these lines may lead to arguments. At this point the individual's health-care provider may also notice something significant and inquire about it.

Overall, the main effect of a serious relationship with one or more substances is the distortion of the lifestyle of the user as substance use gradually becomes more central in the user's life. At the same time, loved ones' lives are affected. They may perceive these changes better than the substance abuser does, and they may begin to resent the ways in which substance abuse has begun to affect their own life. Under this scenario, human relationships begin to deteriorate.

Commitment

- drinks or uses alone most of the time
- has had significant negative consequences clearly connected to substance abuse, such as legal problems (e.g., DUI arrest or conviction), relationship problems (e.g., conflicts over drinking or using, aggression toward others), and health problems
- experiences significant deterioration in roles and responsibilities at home, at work, and so forth

At the commitment stage, the user's lifestyle has shrunk to the point where it revolves around substance use. Maintaining a supply and having access are primary concerns. Hiding or stashing alcohol or drugs is common as is carrying alcohol or drugs on the user's person or in their car. Meanwhile their commitments to family, marriage, or friendships (other than with fellow users) are either lost altogether, for example through divorce, or slip into a state of alienation. This then becomes the starting point when the newly sober individual in recovery begins repairing these damaged relationships.

BUILDING A RECOVERY LIFESTYLE

The fact that the lifestyle of the substance abuser progressively shrinks (and possibly collapses) is the reason why it becomes necessary after rehab to build (or at least rebuild) a lifestyle that will support recovery. Rehab or treatment, in other words, can be the point of departure for a life-changing transformation. However, absent such a transformative process, relapse is likely.

Broadly speaking there are three areas where this transformation needs to begin: with people (relationships), with places, and with daily routines and favored activities. Together these elements make up the fabric of our lifestyle, and in recovery each needs to change. We will take a look at each in turn. First, however, it's important to note again that this work is best approached collaboratively—as a dialogue between the newly sober individual and his or her loved ones. That's not to say that loved ones should dictate what these lifestyle changes will be or how quickly they must happen. On the other hand, both the newly sober man or woman and his or her loved ones are stakeholders in recovery. Just as substance abuse has affected not only the newly sober but also those close to him or her, so it is that these needed changes should be the result of ongoing communication among the stakeholders.

People

Here are a couple of examples of why making changes in one's social network is critical to recovery.

Eric, age thirty-six, had recently been discharged from a twenty-eight-day rehab for his addiction to heroin, which he had turned to when his doctor refused to continue prescribing the pain medication he'd been increasingly abusing and which had originally been prescribed for a chronic back problem related to his years of work as a welder. Eric also had a history of alcohol abuse as well as some mild use of cocaine. On discharge, though, he was clean from all three substances. He was, at that point, receiving unemployment insurance, having been terminated—ostensibly for lack of work but actually because of excessive absenteeism.

As part of his discharge plan, Eric was attending an outpatient group at a local agency twice a week for an hour and a half each visit.

As the final part of his plan, he made an appointment for individual counseling with a female therapist at the same clinic.

At his initial meeting with the therapist, Eric stated that he was not using heroin. He also stated that he did not find the group sessions particularly useful, as they tended to be unfocused and dominated by two or three members. When asked if he had attended any support groups such as AA or SMART Recovery, he said he had not, adding that he had never felt comfortable in large groups. When the therapist asked if that applied as well to the therapy group he attended, Eric offered a weak response: "Well, in the therapy group I can just sit back and listen, but if I went to AA they'd expect me to talk." The therapist knew this was not so and that members were free to speak or just listen at AA meetings, especially in that geographic area, but she decided not to press the issue at her first meeting with Eric.

When Eric showed up for his second therapy session the following week, he reported that he had not been able to attend his group because of car trouble but that he planned to go the next week. The therapist, however, noted that Eric seemed to have a runny nose that he kept wiping with tissues from a dispenser on a table beside him. When she pointed this out, Eric became obviously uncomfortable and replied rather hesitantly that he was coming down with a cold. While that might have been true, the therapist also knew that a runny nose was a common side effect of snorting cocaine and that Eric in fact had some history of that. She next asked Eric who he'd been spending time with since being discharged from treatment as he had not been attending any support groups. He replied that he had been seeing a few of his old friends but repeated that he had not used heroin. That ended the session.

The next week Eric did not show up for his therapy appointment and he did not answer the phone when a scheduler called to reschedule the appointment. Eric did not have any further contact with the agency, and the therapist reasonably surmised that he had relapsed into cocaine use, heroin use, or possibly both.

Elizabeth, an architectural designer, worked for a firm whose specialty was designing interior workspaces for corporations. It was a lucrative profession, and as part of her work she needed to meet with clients often, going to initial meetings to discuss needs, developing and approving plans, then supervising the final installation. This was, understandably, a highly social job that required frequent working lunches and dinners—and wine or cocktails were often a part of that work and social scene.

Elizabeth's mother had been an alcoholic who also suffered from depression. Elizabeth described her as a "quiet alcoholic" who would drink and isolate herself from the family. In addition, Elizabeth had a brother who she believed also had a drinking problem. In her opinion it was shame and stigma that prevented the family from ever talking openly about these issues. She had never married, although one long engagement had ended abruptly when her fiancé announced he had fallen in love with an old high school sweetheart.

After ten very successful years on the job, Elizabeth was elevated to the status of partner. At that point, however, she also had developed a significant drinking problem. She drank every day: at working meetings, after work at home, or (most days) both. She preferred wine with meals but scotch at home. Her daily routine included pouring a large scotch over ice as soon as she got home to her comfortable urban condo. She would then slip into comfortable and familiar clothes and watch the news for half an hour or so in her comfortable lounge chair. Because she ate out in restaurants so often, Elizabeth preferred simple meals at home, either things she could make easily for herself or salads to go from a local supermarket. She would then go on to have two or three more scotches, which she would sip slowly, before retiring for the night. However, she did not sleep well and would often wake up around 2 a.m. and not be able to get back to sleep. She attributed this to the stress of her job (as opposed to her drinking), and when she told her doctor about it, the doctor prescribed a sleep aid that Elizabeth began to take most nights.

As stable and settled as her lifestyle was, Elizabeth had recently learned that she might be in trouble. At an annual physical her doctor had told her that her blood work had come back "a bit worrisome" with respect to her liver function and asked about her drinking. When Elizabeth explained about her mother and brother and also about how much of a role drinking played in her own life, the doctor made three suggestions: first, try to stop drinking altogether for six months, at which time they would repeat the liver function test; second, see a counselor the doctor recommended; and third, consider attending one of the Women for Sobriety meetings being held in the area, which she could find on the internet.

One of the outcomes of Elizabeth's first counseling session was a realization of just how isolated she really was. Despite all of the work-related social contact she had and some social-network friends she had through Facebook, she spent hardly any time face to face with other women other than during the occasional Friday happy hour or over drinks to celebrate a successful project. Moreover, the women she did socialize with at times all drank (though she didn't know how much).

What Eric and Elizabeth, despite their outward differences, had in common was that their social networks were ones that were more inclined to support substance use than sobriety. And it was clear that if either were to pursue abstinence and recovery from substance use, that would need to change. When newly sober individuals hear this, however, their initial reaction is anxiety. Does this mean they have to give up all their old friends? How can they do that? And who would they replace them with? The underlying fear is of becoming socially isolated.

Modifying Your Social Network

Humans are, of course, social animals, and all but very few of us need and seek out social contact. Therefore, even if a newly sober person is able to recognize that their current network of friends and associates is one that tends to support substance use, it is not an easy thing to change that. In this effort, loved ones can play an important role.

Looking back on the examples of Eric and Elizabeth, their reality as newly sober persons reflected complementary challenges. Eric had an existing social network; the problem was that most of these men drank and smoked pot regularly, and a few liked to snort or smoke cocaine on occasion (even if they did not use heroin). Obviously, returning to this social network after treatment represented a significant risk of relapse for Eric.

The situation that Eric faced is also true for most teenage substance abusers who enter treatment. Adolescents by and large are tribal at their developmental stage. They form an identity in part based on the peer group they gravitate toward. These groups are evident in every high school in America. They include the "scholars" (sometimes referred to as "nerds"), "jocks" who excel at sports (and who might also be scholars), "outcasts" who are not part of the social mainstream, "druggies" (no further explanation needed), and "queers" of various sexual orientations. Being an accepted member of one of these groups becomes the foundation for their identity, which in turn can become a template for their future. A teen discharged from a substance-abuse program—no matter how well he or she did and regardless of their stated intention to stay clean and sober—is very likely to return to their old peer group on returning home. This accounts in large part for the high rate of relapse among teenage substance abusers.[1]

In Eric's case there were two most likely explanations for what appeared to be a relapse. On the one hand, on discharge from treatment he may not have been truly committed to abstinence as the best goal. He may have been ambivalent about this, as discussed earlier, and contemplated taking the risk that he could successfully moderate or control his use. Alternatively, like most younger people, he might have simply succumbed to social pressure. He might have found it too daunting to exchange his existing social network, which supported substance abuse, for one that supported recovery.

In contrast, Elizabeth's challenge was a bit different. It was true that much of her social contact tended to revolve around drinking, but it was also true that Elizabeth did not have much of an active social network. In many ways her lifestyle mirrored that of her mother, the quiet alcoholic who spent much of her time alone, drinking. Therefore, what Elizabeth faced was the challenge of *creating* a social network that could support the goal of abstinence from alcohol.

Creating a Social Network

The purpose of this exercise is to guide the newly sober man or woman in reflecting on his or her existing social network and then thinking about how they might go about changing that. A common barrier in this respect is the way that substance abuse tends to skew a person's social network over time. Many people with substance-abuse disorders state that before moving from the low-risk zone of alcohol or drug use further along the substance-use spectrum into the mild, moderate, or even severe zones, they had a more diverse social network; in other words, they had friends and associates who might be nonusers as well as low-risk users. However, over time they drifted toward a social network that tended to reflect their own use. For many this meant pretty much abandoning their old friends and substituting ones who drank or used.

This trend confirms the old adage "Birds of a feather flock together." However, when it comes to substance use, this trend becomes a trap—and one that takes some effort to escape.

Table 6.1 may be helpful in guiding the newly sober through this challenge. It can be helpful to share this with a loved one—not so that the loved one should dictate the outcome but rather so that both can grasp the challenge and perhaps share thoughts about directions to pursue.

As you can see, the exercise is divided into three parts so let's discuss each of these parts separately.

People Who Supported My Substance Use.   This part of the exercise is usually the easiest place to begin. Newly sober readers who reflect on this often are able to see just how their social network changed over time, along with their substance use. The change usually begins

Table 6.1. Lifestyle Contract: Building New Relationships

People Who Supported My Substance Use	People Who Can Support My Recovery	How Can I Build Relationships with a Supportive Social Network?

with gradually avoiding friends and associates who don't drink or use drugs at all and gravitating toward those who drink or use a little, then eventually toward those who are regular users. The last stage also tends to be the social network at the time the substance abuser enters treatment or rehab. AA historically has referred to the people of this social network as "slippery" people because associating with them often and understandably leads to a relapse. Despite that obvious reality, letting go of these relationships may not be easy. For one thing, they may be the only friends the substance abuser has left at this time. They may also be the ones who initiate contact once the newly sober person returns home. And in some cases, they may even be coworkers or associates. That was pretty much the case for both Eric and Elizabeth. As Elizabeth explained to the counselor she met with, she was hard-pressed to think of women that she met with who did not drink, yet she understood that if she was to follow her doctor's advice and not drink at all for six months she would need to either avoid those women altogether (an idea she did not relish) or else come up with some reasonable excuse for not drinking.

There are two social situations in particular that it would be wise for the newly sober person to think about and decide how they might go about dealing with, and the first has to do with close friends who drink or use drugs on a more or less frequent basis. For example, Brian, age thirty, had a longstanding habit of meeting friends at a sports bar to watch Monday Night Football. While not all of these friends drank heavily, they all drank. Meanwhile, Brian had been drinking heavily since his freshman year in college to the point where he went to his doctor because of abdominal pain, underwent testing, and was told he had an inflamed pancreas and would need to alter his diet, and stop drinking immediately, or risk slipping into pancreatitis, a serious health condition.

Brian's friends were not aware of his diagnosis, and he explained to the counselor that he felt it would be too embarrassing to admit to the truth of his problem and explain why he could not drink. Nevertheless, the counselor told Mark that it was just too risky for him to go to sports bars. "That would be like a gambling addict telling me," the counselor remarked, "that he wants to go to a casino to meet friends because he likes the restaurants!"

In cases like Brian's, honesty is actually the best policy. The best course of action is to step up and say that your doctor has advised you to stop drinking. True friends can accept (and respect) such honesty.

There is no need to go into any lengthy explanations of your drinking (or using) history or all of the details for why you have decided to stop drinking. It's sufficient, for example, to say there is a history of a certain illness in your family such that you've been advised by your doctor to not drink (or use drugs of any kind). You then need to decide where you want to meet these friends moving forward. More about that later.

The other risky social situation concerns family members who drink or use a lot, and the riskiest situation usually has to do with family gatherings. Jeanna, who was in rehab for alcohol and prescription tranquilizer abuse, told her group that most everyone in her family had a drinking problem or a drug problem but that no one ever talked about it even though a cousin had recently overdosed on heroin and nearly died. One of her main concerns was how she was going to cope when the family got together for a holiday or a birthday as was their habit. Others in the group expressed similar concerns. They then did some brainstorming and came up with the following ideas:

- Minimize the number of times Jeanna went to such occasions as well as how long she stayed there.
- Go to a recovery fellowship, make a few friends, and have one of those friends call Jeanna at an arranged time and give her an excuse to leave.
- Bring a sober friend or supportive loved one to such events and leave at an agreed-upon time, using any agreed-upon excuse.
- Try honesty: just tell the family that she has gone through treatment and is not drinking at all.

Having to deal with social situations like the above is common among newly sober men and women, and it can be awkward or even intimidating. It may take some practice as well as some courage. However, the support of loved ones who are stakeholders in recovery, as well as the help that comes from reaching out to others who are also pursuing recovery, can make these situations manageable. In the worst-case scenario, it may be necessary for the newly sober person to avoid some social contacts entirely if these contacts represent a threat to recovery.

People Who Can Support My Recovery.   The most obvious answer to who these people are is the men and women who choose to participate in a recovery fellowship that supports abstinence. That was the reason Elizabeth's doctor brought up Women for Sobriety and also why Eric's counselor asked him about attending AA. If associates who drink or use drugs are "slippery," then clearly those whose goal is abstinence represent solid ground. The fact that there is AA—but also alternatives to AA—suggests that there really should be no excuses for giving a recovery fellowship a try (other than ambivalence about wanting to abstain). Even social anxiety can be addressed with the help of a counselor or online meetings.

Some people ask if it is possible to build a supportive social network by building new friendships, or rekindling old ones, without partaking in a recovery fellowship. This question has been the subject of research.[2] The researchers divided a sample of men and women with alcohol abuse disorders into two treatment groups. The first group was asked to attend AA meetings as a means of staying sober. The second group was also asked to attend AA but was told in addition that they should try to increase the time they spent with any nondrinking friends or family members that they knew. The results were informative: spending added time with sober friends could help support abstinence but not nearly as much as attending AA. In addition, the men and women in the study reported that they were able to find no more than one or two nonusing people in their social network. So the answer to this question is that it's fine to spend time with sober friends but that may not be easy, and participating in a recovery fellowship such as AA, SMART Recovery, or Women for Sobriety is much more powerful.

When working on this part of the exercise, the newly sober person should keep the above in mind. Essentially, doing both makes sense. However, it would seem to be apparent that participating in a fellowship in which members are pursuing a common goal has advantages over spending time with friends or family members who are sober and with whom the newly sober person may not feel comfortable talking about their goal of abstinence.

How Can I Build Relationships with a Supportive Social Network? Building new relationships—especially relationships that will support recovery—from the ground up can be difficult. However, some avenues are easier than others, beginning again with looking into and trying out one or more of the recovery fellowships we've reviewed. The newly sober person can begin by going online and learning something about each fellowship. Fortunately, all these fellowships publish a great deal of information that is either free on the internet or available at very low cost. Next, the newly sober person can take the step of attending a couple of different meetings. The words "a couple" are important because while all of these fellowships follow their own unique format, in reality none are so highly centralized that every meeting will be identical. It's important to keep this in mind and therefore to feel free to shop around a bit to find meetings where you feel most comfortable. AA in particular has a diversity of meetings, especially in urban and suburban areas. Also, in AA the newcomer is often invited to simply "be there"—to listen and observe without feeling obligated to participate more than that.

The next step in using a recovery fellowship to support abstinence is to gradually get more involved: to speak up at times, to socialize before and after meetings, and to gradually build new relationships. Building friendships outside meetings is also a part of this process. This takes time, of course, but it can also be the foundation for recovery.

MOVING FORWARD

Breaking free of destructive relationships and working toward building supportive ones may be the single most important component of a recovery lifestyle. It can mark the start of nothing less than a personal transformation. But it is not the only component. In the next chapter we will look at more of the building blocks of a recovery lifestyle.

・ *7* ・

Creating a Recovery Lifestyle

Part 2: Places, Routines, and Interests

𝒯he voyage to recovery continues across what is best thought of as the open water that follows rehab or other formal treatment, and it is a challenge that should not be underestimated. In this chapter we extend the challenge to include creating a new lifestyle that will support recovery as opposed to substance use. The fact is that as a person moves along the substance-use spectrum from low-risk use to mild, moderate, or even severe substance abuse, his or her lifestyle essentially shrinks to the point where it revolves around getting and using his or her substance of abuse. That kind of lifestyle is highly limited. Former nonusing friends are gradually abandoned. Activities that once were a source of enjoyment drift away. And life comes to revolve around routines and even rituals that support substance use. In contrast, creating and living a sober lifestyle can be nothing less than transformative, as many men and women who enjoy such a lifestyle can attest.

PLACES AND ROUTINES

Sarah evolved into a heavy drinker slowly but steadily over a period of many years. It started in college, where like many of her classmates she partied on a regular basis. Mostly these parties involved alcohol and cannabis, but occasionally partygoers would add pills to the mix. There were times when Sarah swallowed pills she didn't even know the names of after getting drunk, and more than once she passed out only to wake up the next morning in bed beside a male student she did not even know.

75

After graduating Sarah got an entry-level job in finance and then pursued a master's degree part time. She was now a mid-level executive in a large financial management firm and doing well, at least in terms of income. She was divorced with two college-age children, a son and a daughter, who had long rotated residency between their parents but who both spent little time at either place since going off to college. These days Sarah's weekly schedule typically included grabbing a light dinner in one of three restaurants, especially after a long day at the office. She had developed a taste for martinis and would usually consume two while she ate and read the news on her tablet. On getting home she would pour a glass of white wine, change into pajamas, and watch the news or a favored show or two on TV. She'd usually mute the TV for a brief phone call to a man she'd been dating for the past year. She liked him, thought he was bright, and generally enjoyed his company though she'd also pretty much decided that she was not interested in living with him much less marrying a second time.

Over the past year or so Sarah had experienced trouble sleeping (which, like most people in the mild-to-moderate substance-use zone, she did not attribute to her drinking). After a consultation with her doctor—during which she did not disclose her fondness for martinis—she was prescribed a sleep aid, which she'd been taking nightly for the better part of nine months. When her doctor suggested cutting back on the sleep aid, Sarah tried but found that made her sleeplessness worse, so her doctor relented and agreed to continue the prescription but with the condition that she not increase the dosage.

Then after an annual physical, the doctor told Sarah that she was prediabetic. At this point the drinking came out, though Sarah still downplayed it. Nevertheless, the doctor strongly recommended that Sarah either severely limit her alcohol intake or quit entirely, at least for the time being while they monitored her health. Sarah agreed to this, but when it came to actually doing it, she stumbled badly. First, she found it very difficult to resist going to her favorite restaurants, which had become part of the fabric of her lifestyle. And when she did go, she found it impossible to decline the martini that her server was ready to deliver. Similarly, not having a couple of glasses of wine while relaxing and watching TV was another challenge. The bottom line was that after six months Sarah had not made much progress at all on her doctor's recommendation, and subsequent tests revealed that her condition appeared to be getting worse, to the point where medication might be needed.

Sarah is not an untypical example by any means. We are all creatures of habit. Think for a moment about your own daily routines, from the time you wake until the time you go to bed. How easy would it be for you to alter one of these routines? This is a good exercise for both the newly sober and his or her loved ones to try. It will give both an appreciation for just how much of a challenge this aspect of building a recovery lifestyle can be.

Martin is another example. A former marine who served six tours of duty in Mideast wars, he had been diagnosed with a traumatic brain injury plus post-traumatic stress disorder (PTSD) following an attack on his post and placed on disability. He took medication but attended the group therapy sessions that his doctor at the VA hospital recommended rather inconsistently. Like his father and grandfather, Martin had always been something of a drinker, but after his diagnosis he soon became a daily consumer of beer and, later, cannabis. He was married and had a son who was a senior in high school. Martin was glad that his son had expressed an interest in pursuing a career as an electrician rather than in the military.

Martin had been married to Lucy for twenty years and considered the marriage solid despite his repeated absences and now his medical and psychiatric diagnoses, which had resulted in a chronic, low-grade depression in addition to his substance abuse. Unlike many men who suffer from PTSD, Martin was not violent. Instead, his lifestyle had come to revolve around the basement of his home. It was a walk-out basement that had a heater as well as a large, flat-screen TV and a small refrigerator that Martin kept filled with beer. He enjoyed watching sports while drinking and getting high on cannabis. The basement also included a small work area where Martin engaged in his one hobby: building small birdhouses that he then sometimes sold at a local flea market. He'd found that he could make enough money that way to pay for his beer and cannabis, so he did not need to use any of his disability income for that.

There were two consequences of his substance use that proved to be a problem for Martin. First, he was pretty much an absentee member of the family—which his wife and son both regularly complained about. They also were unhappy that Martin was so lax about pursuing treatment for his PTSD other than taking an antidepressant. Second, his family had a history of liver disease. His grandfather had died from cirrhosis, and the family suspected that a failing liver, along with heart disease, had played a role in his father's death at fifty-one. While Martin tried to avoid talking about this, his doctor (who essentially knew at least about Martin's drinking) often did, as a warning, as did Martin's son, who more than once commented that he was not eager to be a fatherless son.

Things came to a head for Martin when he began to experience the kind of chest discomfort and breathing difficulty that he remembered his father having. When he experienced acute chest pain in the middle of the night, his son drove him to the emergency room at the VA hospital, where he was evaluated and admitted for angina. Further testing revealed coronary artery disease, which the doctors attributed partly to genetics but mostly to Martin's drinking and daily pot smoking. This scared him, and when he was discharged (with additional medication) he was told he needed to stop both. This information was also shared with Martin's wife and son, and although Martin agreed to this remedy, like Sarah, he found it very difficult to follow through.

Martin's case presents a good example of how a collaborative approach to recovery can work. Left to his own devices Martin would no doubt have struggled greatly to make changes in his lifestyle—places and routines—that could support staying clean and sober even though not doing so would clearly put his health at risk. Instead, Martin allowed his son and wife to be included in discussions with his doctors, and because the full extent of his alcohol and cannabis use came out in those discussions, they were able collectively to come up with a plan that could literally make the difference between life and death for Martin. Here are some of the elements of that plan:

- Martin would no longer shop for beer or contact his cannabis supplier. Instead, his son would purchase a limited amount of nonalcoholic beer that Martin could have every week.
- The basement refrigerator would be retired. The nonalcoholic beer would be kept in a refrigerator upstairs.
- The wide-screen television in the basement, along with Martin's recliner, would be moved to a spare bedroom upstairs.

- Martin could continue with his bird house hobby, but his son could choose to work with him at times to learn the skill. They would then sell the houses they made together.
- Martin would meet individually with a substance-abuse counselor at the VA hospital every two weeks.

The above recovery plan worked for Martin. To his credit he took his family's concerns and his doctors' warnings to heart and was willing to work collaboratively with them.

Sarah's situation was somewhat more challenging as she did not have either a spouse or children living with her that she could readily collaborate with. In her case she chose to work with a therapist to collaboratively make changes in places and routines so as to create lifestyle changes that would support her desire to stay sober. To begin, she had to admit that as much as she liked her three favorite restaurants, there were others close enough to her condo that she could replace them with. In fact, to her pleasant surprise she found two that she liked even better! Meeting weekly with her therapist, she also was able to open up about some other issues, such as how isolated her life had become outside work, how she really desired more contact with her children but was hesitant to ask for it, and how it was she and not her boyfriend who maintained the distance in their relationship. Some of these issues contributed to the limited lifestyle that Sarah lived, and none of them was easy to work on. But with the support of her therapist she chipped away at them. One additional change she made in terms of places and routines was to join a fitness center. She began going there three days a week after work instead of heading straight to a restaurant or home for her TV and wine. She soon found that exercising, losing a bit of weight, sleeping better, and feeling more energetic made her less interested in drinking wine at night. There were now nights when she did not drink at all; and on those increasingly rare occasions when she did drink, it tended to be one glass rather that two or three.

PLACES AND ROUTINES THAT INCLUDE LOVED ONES

The situations that newly sober people often report as particularly challenging are those places and routines associated with substance use that include family members. They are often reluctant to address these—or change them—in part for fear of offending any family members who would likely be part of such a scenario. Beyond that, they may fear becoming essentially an outcast by defying the family culture. One example is Helen, age sixty-five, who with her husband Ted had sold their home a year earlier and moved to a retirement community. They loved the warm weather as well as the company that was available at the large clubhouse that was a feature of the community.

Both Ted and Helen had long enjoyed an afternoon cocktail and sometimes two; however, since moving and getting involved in the new community, their drinking had steadily increased along the substance-use spectrum to the point where between clubhouse gatherings and frequent, informal, social engagements at home, they were now consuming twenty or more cocktails every week. This is substantially more than what is considered low-risk drinking by national standards. In fact, that level of drinking put both Ted and Helen in the excessive drinking category[1] or what would qualify as at least a mild alcohol-use disorder. Of course because they had slid into this category slowly, and partly through the new drinking norms that some of their new friends observed, they were not cognizant of being in any danger. However, Helen was a cancer survivor and Ted had undergone surgery to have two stents installed in his heart. Although alcohol abuse is a risk factor for cancer survivors,[2] it was actually Ted who first experienced symptoms that related to his increased drinking. The first of these was insomnia. He'd never had trouble sleeping soundly, but over the past six months he'd found himself unable to sleep through the night. He'd wake up in the wee hours and then not be able to get back to sleep. This led to him being groggy and lethargic the next day. Helen mentioned the drinking, but Ted dismissed that in favor of thinking it was just a sign of aging. But then he experienced tightness in his chest. That motivated him to see a doctor, who did a thorough assessment (taking into account Ted's drinking as well as an echocardiogram), after which he informed Ted that his symptoms were an early sign of a potential return of the circulatory problem that had led to the stents. He strongly advised Ted to either stop drinking or limit himself to no more than five cocktails per week. He also scheduled a follow-up for six weeks later.

This presented both Helen and Ted with a challenge. Not only would following the doctor's advice mean significant changes in people, places, and routines for Ted, it also had implications for Helen. It would mean making changes in their social interactions and also in their routines at home. If Ted were to try to limit himself to no more than five drinks a week, what would that mean for Helen? Making changes in their clubhouse activities together was one thing, but what about their longstanding routine of the daily afternoon cocktail or two?

Despite their having a strong and long marriage, Helen had a hard time coming to terms with the new limitation. For one thing, her own drinking had increased over the past year—and then there was the issue of giving up her daily afternoon cocktails. At first Ted tried reassuring her that it would be okay if he had only the five drinks while she could have as many as she wanted. With respect to their new social network, they agreed the best policy was to step up and share the results of Ted's exam as well as his doctor's advice. That could mean spending less time at the clubhouse or even foregoing activities that included drinking. For the most part they found that their new social circle accepted Ted drinking very little, but they did not see any need to cut down on their own drinking. Helen admitted that she found this situation frustrating as she would want to drink more on these occasions while at the same time support Ted by not presenting him with temptation.

After a month the results were that Ted had substantially reduced his alcohol consumption but was still beyond the five-drink limit. He'd avoided talking to Helen about his struggle, but as his follow-up appointment approached, he felt an obligation to bring it up. Helen's initial reaction was not all that positive. She said that she had limited herself to a single cocktail a day, sometimes two, and had assumed that Ted would just follow the doctor's advice. Ted then responded that he was aware of what Helen was doing but that it was just too difficult for him to completely break a routine that had been such a central part of their lives for so many years. He said he now believed they needed to make a significant change if he was to reliably reduce his drinking.

They settled on two new routines. First, they agreed that three days a week they would substitute a walk along the community's many walking paths for the usual cocktails. And as a compromise they also agreed that Helen could indulge in a cocktail in another part of the condo while Ted pursued his hobby of reading history and engaging in online chats with fellow history buffs in another room that served as an informal office and guest room. This meant that they would not be sharing cocktails as often as they were accustomed to, but they agreed that it was a necessary change.

In general it takes roughly ninety days for a new habit or routine to begin to feel comfortable and replace a former routine. During this initial ninety-day period, both Ted and Helen admitted that there were times they felt uncomfortable and yearned for a return to their old ritual. But because they agreed that it was important for Ted's health, they stuck with it. In time Helen came to agree that it was best for her, as a cancer survivor, as well.

THE PLACES AND ROUTINES WORKSHEET

People who want to strengthen their recovery and who also recognize the role that places and routines can play in it can benefit from having something concrete to use as a guide. Table 7.1 will be helpful in this regard.

Table 7.1.   **Places and Routines Worksheet**

Places Associated with My Substance Use	Places That Could Support My Recovery
Routines Associated with My Substance Use	Routines That Could Support My Recovery

Like the exercise on people, this worksheet provides a vehicle for a fruitful dialogue between the newly sober man or woman and his or her loved ones. The challenge of making significant changes in one's lifestyle, despite the best of intentions, can at the outset seem like an almost insurmountable mountain to climb. Like Ted and Helen and the other examples we've looked at, this can be a lot easier if it's approached as a joint venture. I often suggest that the newly sober along with his or her loved ones think of themselves as fellow crew members on the voyage to recovery. This almost always leads to an experience that is ultimately rewarding to all who participate since the changes they make often benefit everyone concerned, as was the case for Ted and Helen. When working on this exercise keep the following in mind:

- Be creative. Think outside the box about how changes in where you spend your time and your daily routines can potentially benefit everyone.
- Think of healthy new routines that can be shared. Don't be afraid to break out of the mold together.
- Support each other's efforts to make these lifestyle changes. Be each other's best cheerleader!

ACTIVITIES

We know that as a substance-abuse problem progresses along the substance-use spectrum, the user's lifestyle gradually shrinks. At first these changes—which are actually losses—may not be so noticeable. As a person moves from low-risk use to a mild-use disorder, for example, he or she may simply devote less time to activities once looked forward to and that once played an important part in their lifestyle. Then over time they may abandon some of these activities completely. In the case of Ted, while he'd been a lifetime history buff, he'd pretty much given up his online chats since his and Helen's drinking had come to play a larger part in their daily life. So it goes with substance abuse. As it progresses, lives shrink, potentially to the point where life literally revolves around obtaining and using the substance that the user eventually becomes a slave to. Reversing this process is a key ingredient of recovery. If you ask an adolescent addict what he or she enjoys doing, they will typically shrug. "Get high," they might say. This is the case for any alcoholic, who may manage to get to and from work but whose life remains centered on a state of inebriation.

This issue of activities is another instance where newly sober individuals and their loved ones can benefit from concrete guidance that can also be a vehicle to spur a useful dialogue leading to collaborative changes. Table 7.2 will be useful for this purpose.

Table 7.2.   Activities Worksheet

Activities Lost or Abandoned Because of Substance Use	Activities I Might Resume or Try Out

Ian, at age thirty-three, was a professor of chemistry. Never married, he had been dating Jennifer, a fellow professor, steadily for the past year or so. Divorced, Jennifer had a nine-year-old son and was fortunate to have parents who lived fairly close by and who loved nothing more than seeing their grandson. Though he'd never thought much about fatherhood, Ian enjoyed the boy's company and found him to be bright and cheerful. While neither Ian nor Jennifer had yet been awarded tenure, the positions of both were secure—at least, they had been until recently.

Ian had been athletic his entire life. Raised in upper New England, he virtually grew up on ski slopes and ice rinks. In addition he was an avid runner. That all changed, however, and suddenly, when he hit an ice patch while careening down an expert slope and badly injured his back, eventually requiring surgery to fuse three vertebrae. That ended both his skiing and his running career but also left Ian with chronic, severe pain that was initially treated with pain medication. The problem was that after taking the medication—an opioid—for six months, Ian found himself getting extremely uncomfortable, even agitated, without it. His surgeon referred him to a pain clinic, but that didn't help much. The surgeon reluctantly agreed to continue the medication, but insisted on a lower dose. Ian did the best he could, but eventually he found that the best way to relieve his pain was taking the medication along with a few shots of the whiskey his father had favored.

Jennifer knew that Ian had been given pain medication, but she was not aware that he'd developed a tolerance to it—and indeed, a dependency on it. He also limited his drinking to when he was home alone at night. In this way he was able to maintain his academic load as well as work on two grants for submission, which was important to his case for tenure.

Things went along like that until Ian happened across a news article describing how people were able to obtain prescription opioids without a prescription over the internet through what were essentially pill factories operated by shady businesses. He found himself mulling this over for a few weeks, but then relented, looked up the article again, and with remarkable ease was able to connect to such a site. Soon he was purchasing and using opioids daily in greater doses than ever. On top of that he also continued to drink whiskey on those nights he wasn't seeing Jennifer.

It took about six months before Ian's work at the university began to slip. He began to cancel classes once or twice a week. Then he took to recording some lessons and having his classes watch them online. None of his colleagues said anything, but Ian knew that the chemistry department was like a small town and that others were surely aware of the changes. His main concern was that this would include his department head and the dean. Still he continued taking both the pills and the liquor.

The crisis struck one night when Jennifer tried repeatedly to contact Ian by text and phone but got no response. That was not at all like him. Since she had a key to his apartment, she decided to drop her son at her parents' and take a quick run over to check on him. She arrived to find Ian on the floor in the living room beside his sofa, unconscious, an open pill container and bottle of whiskey on a side table. She was both shocked and alarmed. Ian, it turned out, had come perilously close to overdosing on a potentially lethal combination of opioids and alcohol. It was fortunate that Jennifer had found him and had the good sense to call 911.

Ian's recovery began with his detox in the hospital, followed by a visit to his regular physician. It was at the visit that his doctor confronted Ian frankly. He said he was going to prescribe Suboxone to help Ian come off the prescription opioids. But then he added, "You also need to quit the booze. If you don't I can bet that you will relapse on the prescription drugs." He then referred Ian to a therapist he knew and added that he strongly recommended Ian start attending AA meetings. "Don't kid yourself," he said, "you're going to need all the help you can get. You're addicted to opioids, and from what I gather, your father may have been an alcoholic, and you have the same genes. Research shows that one can easily lead to the other."

Ian then faced the greatest challenge of his life and one that would literally mean the difference between success and failure in his career, between a good relationship and isolation, and possibly even between life and death. To his credit he chose recovery. With respect to adding activities that would support his recovery as opposed to continued substance abuse, here is what Ian chose to do:

- He took to using the university's athletic center, which featured a pool and was available to faculty, for exercise that didn't cause much pain.
- He started attending two different men's AA meetings each week, one during the week and one on the weekend. Despite his initial expectation that he would not be able to relate to the men he'd meet there, he was pleased to find that they were down to earth and supportive of his need to quit drinking even if they did not share his problem with opioids.
- The therapist Ian saw recommended he look into trying mindfulness meditation, a technique that had been found to be effective in pain control.[3] Ian did so with the goal of eventually weaning himself off the medication, and in combination with

physical therapy, over time he found that he was able to make progress in that regard.

- He and Jennifer joined an outdoor adventure club with a focus on the environment, including nature walks and nonstrenuous hikes. Her son joined them on many of these occasions, and Ian found that with the aid of hiking sticks he was able to enjoy the hikes.
- Ian reached out to and connected with Jennifer's son on some joint ventures, including seeing some movies together, spending time at a model railroad store that featured room-size model setups, and taking in some university sporting events.

PURSUING TRANSFORMATION

The issues we've covered in this chapter and the aspects of recovery they involve tend to blend into one another. Changes in people, places, and routines can easily spill over into changes in activities. Ian's case and the others discussed here are good examples of this. The common denominator is that recovery, if it is to be resilient and robust, requires changes in lifestyle as much as it requires a motivation to stay clean and sober. Finally, as represented in many of the above examples, many of these lifestyle changes can be effectively approached collaboratively between a newly sober person and his or her loved ones, and they can be mutually satisfying and beneficial. As mentioned earlier, the pursuit of a new lifestyle can literally become a transformative experience.

· 8 ·

Double Trouble

Substance Abuse and Mental Illness

ALCOHOL USE AND ITS RELATION
TO MENTAL ILLNESS

This is an important issue that has not received the attention it deserves. It's also one that the newly sober person and his or her loved ones need to know about in order to work collaboratively in the interest of promoting a robust recovery. Lack of knowledge in this area—a lack of understanding or failure to treat a mental illness—can place the voyage to recovery in serious jeopardy.

In order to gain some understanding of this issue, the National Institute on Alcohol Abuse and Alcoholism (NIAAA) funded a major national survey on alcohol use and its relation to mental illness.[1] The survey was designed to reflect the entire U.S. population. Data were collected through personal interviews. In all, 20,291 people ages eighteen and older were interviewed. The interview was aimed at collecting information on the participants' experiences during the previous year. Confidentiality was guaranteed to facilitate getting accurate information.

This survey focused primarily on men and women whose drinking fell into one of two zones on the drinking spectrum that we reviewed earlier: moderate alcohol-use disorders and severe alcohol-use disorders. In collecting data that was supposed to be representative of the entire population, they necessarily also interviewed men and women who had neither a significant drinking problem nor a mental illness. In the interviews, information was collected on how much the individual drank as well as whether they had ever been diagnosed with one of a number of psychiatric illnesses. The researchers were not so much interested in whether the individuals being interviewed were in treatment for either a drinking problem or a mental illness so much as they wanted to gain insight into how many people had

- both a mental illness and a substance-use disorder (a so-called dual-diagnosis, or co-occurring disorder);
- either a mental illness or a substance-use disorder;
- neither a mental illness nor a substance-use disorder.

Let's take a look at what this extensive research yielded. The study authors not only reported simple percentages but also presented their data in a unique way: in terms of the odds of having a particular mental illness if your drinking pattern fell into one of the above two categories as opposed to not having either of these drinking problems. We can best look at the results in table form (see table 8.1).

Table 8.1. NIAAA National Survey

Mental Illness	Odds: Moderate Alcohol Disorder	Odds: Severe Alcohol Disorder
Depression	1.1 to 1	3.9 to 1
Anxiety	1.7 to 1	2.6 to 1
PTSD	1.5 to 1	2.2 to 1
Schizophrenia	1.9 to 1	3.8 to 1

How should we understand the data in this table? It tells us, for example, that men and women whose drinking placed them at the moderate alcohol-use disorder zone on the drinking spectrum and people who had no alcohol-use disorder had about equal chances of having suffered from depression in the previous year (a 1.1 to 1 ratio). In other words, this level of drinking did not appear to pose a greater risk than average for depression.

In a stark contrast, look at those men and women with a severe drinking problem. They were almost four times as likely to have experienced depression in the previous year than those men and women with no drinking problem (a 3.9 to 1 ratio).

As for anxiety disorders, there is a direct relationship between where someone is on the drinking spectrum and the likelihood that they will have one of these disorders. For example, the 1.7 to 1 ratio for anxiety disorders means that people with a moderate alcohol-use disorder are 70 percent more likely to suffer from an anxiety disorder than those whose drinking pattern falls somewhere short of that. And if they move into the severe alcohol-use disorder zone, they are more than twice as likely to have an anxiety disorder than someone who drinks less.

Moving on to PTSD, we once again see a relationship between drinking and PTSD such that heavier drinkers are more likely than moderate drinkers to suffer from this debilitating disorder. The same is true to an even greater extent for the diagnosis of schizophrenia: the heavy drinker is much more likely to have that additional diagnosis.

What does all this data mean? Does it mean that drinking causes anxiety, depression, PTSD, or even schizophrenia? Probably not, because it does not make sense that drinking by itself could cause such a diverse range of mental illnesses. What it does suggest, however, are several things:

- A significant number (though by no means all) of men and women who seek treatment for a drinking problem, or decide to turn to AA or an alternative recovery fellowship for support, suffer from some form of mental illness in addition to their drinking problem.
- Men and women with more-severe drinking problems are even more likely to have an additional mental illness. It is possible that their drinking has made their mental illness worse or, alternatively, that they have turned to drinking as a means of self-medicating their mental illness.
- The best approach would be to recognize the existence of this dual-diagnosis (or co-occurring disorder) population and make their recovery easier by encouraging them to treat both their mental illness and drinking problem at the same time.

SELF-MEDICATION

The idea that some people who end up with a significant drinking problem may have used alcohol or drugs such as cannabis initially in an effort to relieve symptoms of a mental illness is worth a further look. It's well known, for example, that men and women who suffer from PTSD—

such as soldiers exposed to chronic stress as a result of deployment to a combat zone—also abuse alcohol and drugs, especially cannabis. They may indeed have turned to alcohol (or cannabis) as a means of relieving symptoms such as anxiety, edginess, poor sleep, and even flashbacks.

If we reflect on it for a moment, it seems clear that a number of the individuals we've discussed so far may well have qualified for having both a mental illness and a substance-abuse problem. It's no secret that men and women have, for generations, turned to substance use in a unilateral effort to mitigate anxiety, depression, mood swings, and even hallucinations. Before the advent of modern psychiatry there were really no options. Indeed, even Bill Wilson, cofounder of AA, acknowledged his longstanding struggle with depression.[2]

The newly sober man or woman reading this book along with his or her loved ones would be wise to take some time to reflect on this issue as it may apply to him or her. There are two broad areas to consider when contemplating whether a mental health issue may coexist with a substance-abuse issue and if so, what to do about it moving forward. These areas are, respectively, genetics and experience.

THE GENETICS OF SUBSTANCE ABUSE

To begin this discussion, it must be acknowledged that the idea that alcoholism in particular, which has been studied the most, but perhaps more broadly substance-abuse disorders in general, tends to run in families has been well documented by research.[3] Surveys have consistently found that first-degree relatives (parents, siblings, and children) of those who have been treated for alcoholism are two to four times more likely to be alcoholics than the relatives of nonalcoholics.[4] Studies of identical twins in which one is an alcoholic have shown that the other twin has a roughly 50 percent chance of also being an alcoholic.[5]

Information like this should give anyone who has a family member who they either know to have a drinking problem, or who has actually been treated for alcoholism, pause to reflect on their own drinking. While most research has focused on alcoholism, it is probably reasonable to assume that this genetic vulnerability would apply to other substances as well. In other words, the capacity to develop a tolerance—and subsequently a craving—for alcohol could well apply to substances like cannabis, cocaine, and so forth.

As much as this data should be a wake-up call for readers who have a history of substance-use disorders in their family, it is definitely not inevitable that everyone in this situation will develop such problems. Even among identical twins, as noted above, where the genetic risk appears to be greatest, there is also a 50 percent chance that the twin of an alcoholic will not become an alcoholic. The difference will be accounted for largely by whether these individuals heed the warning and either refrain from substance abuse or take care to stay in the low-risk zone. It also will depend on the kind of lifestyle they may have developed and whether that lifestyle also tends to support sobriety, or at least low-risk use.

THE GENETICS OF MENTAL ILLNESS

Researchers have also looked into family patterns relative to mental illness. For example, studies of major depression and bipolar disorder have shown, as in alcoholism, that first-degree relatives of individuals diagnosed with these disorders are indeed at increased risk of developing these disorders as compared to first-degree relatives of those without them.[6]

As for anxiety disorders, researchers have reported that these are one of the more familial diseases, and not only that two-thirds of cases have relatives affected with the same condition but also that the risk to first-degree relatives is approximately three to four times the rate of the general population. And among identical twins, the data tell us that they have a 30–40 percent chance of both having the disorder if one does as opposed to only a 4 percent or less chance among fraternal twins.[7]

All of these studies, combined with the results of the NIAAA survey, point in one direction: substance abuse and mental illness frequently coexist, and men and women may have historically turned to using substances in an effort to manage a mental illness only to end up caught in the web of addiction.

EXPERIENCE, MENTAL ILLNESS,
AND SUBSTANCE ABUSE

While genetics may provide an important warning sign as to whether an individual may be susceptible to developing a mental illness, an addiction, or both, it is by no means the sole indication. The experiences that individuals have must also be taken into account. An obvious example is PTSD. Although it may be the case that some individuals are more genetically vulnerable to developing this disorder, the etiology also requires experience. Examples we all are familiar with is the soldier who must endure multiple tours in a war zone or the individual who survives a plane crash or serious car accident. But there are also those individuals who are exposed to less dramatic but more chronic stress, including children who are raised under the specter of a violent parent and experience the kind of constant anxiety that can eventually lead to depression or PTSD. The same is true for victims of sexual assault or sexual abuse.

Symptoms of PTSD include intermittent depression, "free-floating" anxiety that hangs like a cloud over the individual, hypervigilance (against threats), a heightened startle response, insomnia, and irritability. Some people with PTSD can be violent; others can be suicidal. Given this range of symptoms, it's little wonder that many may be tempted to turn to substances such as alcohol and cannabis, and even heroin, in an effort to dampen their symptoms.

Abigail—or Abby as she was called—was in her junior year of college and doing poorly. She'd been an excellent student throughout high school and a member of the cheerleading squad and volleyball team as well. Nevertheless, she started drinking at age fifteen, in the context of parties, and in short order was stashing liquor in her closet. She also started smoking cannabis, mostly on weekends.

The reasons for Abby's turning to drinking and smoking pot had to do with disturbing symptoms she'd had for a long time—well before she discovered either alcohol or pot. The roots had to do with her father, who was a violent alcoholic and who abused both Abby and her older sister. Whereas Abby's older sister had to endure mostly demeaning verbal abuse, Abby, though younger, was bigger and stronger and was therefore subject to physical abuse as well. Their mother, a nurse, tried to shield them, and fights between her and Abby's father were frequent. But their mother also had to work, often second shift, and so the girls necessarily had to be alone with their father quite a bit. That was when they both started to experience depression, which for Abby was so debilitating at times that she could not bring herself to get out of bed in the morning and so missed school on occasion. Her escape was cheerleading and, while the season lasted, volleyball. In addition she was bright and able to succeed in school despite a less-than-stellar attendance record. Still she was an anxious girl who preferred to spend as much time as possible in her bedroom with the door locked.

The turning point for Abby proved to be an occasion at college, in her freshman year, when she got drunk and high at a party and left with a male student she didn't know. He walked her back to her dorm room, where he attempted to rape her. Abby, despite her condition, was able to fend the student off but then woke up the next day distraught. A friend encouraged Abby to report the attempted rape, but Abby refused, as she was too embarrassed about being drunk and blamed her own poor judgment. But from there on her grades began to slowly decline, and she found herself slipping back into her old pattern of being too depressed to get out of bed on some mornings. At that point she was stashing liquor in her dorm room as well as smoking pot every weekend.

When friends noticed this pattern, as well as Abby's declining grades, they met with her to insist that she seek help through the university's mental health service. Through therapy she was able for the first time to unburden herself about the abuse she'd endured along with a lot of guilt for not having stood up more to her father's abuse of her sister. A year earlier her parents had finally divorced, and though both girls were grateful for that, they were away at college now and had little interest in spending much time back at home.

WHAT WE KNOW ABOUT TREATMENT FOR CO-OCCURRING DISORDERS

Abby had what we are discussing here: a substance-abuse disorder and concurrent mental illness. Although she was not yet an alcoholic, she was on the way. Left to her own devices, which involved drinking and smoking cannabis to deal with her depression and anxiety, she could well have ended up there (as well as flunking out of college).

The treatment that Abby received was consistent with what we know about successfully tackling a co-occurring disorder. This included psychotherapy along with medication. Neither of these, by themselves, is as successful as both used at the same time. Abby was referred by her therapist to a nurse practitioner who assessed her and shared her opinion that depression was the most dominant problem that plagued Abby, and so Abby was prescribed an antidepressant. While the nurse practitioner acknowledged that Abby also suffered from anxiety, the nurse knew that taking antianxiety medications can lead to addiction, and she wanted to avoid that possibility. She also told Abby that drinking would effectively cancel the effects of the antidepressant. Therefore, if the medication was to work, Abby would need to forego alcohol—at least for the foreseeable future while she, the nurse practitioner, and the therapist worked collaboratively. The nurse also told Abby that she was not the only college student who had developed a drinking problem. She was aware of at least one AA meeting on campus that welcomed students, as well as one Women for Sobriety meeting that met in a nearby town. She suggested Abby try reaching out to both for support.

The combination that Abby pursued worked for her, and it can work for many newly sober individuals who are able to face up to their co-occurring mental health issues and have the courage to pursue a dual recovery from both substance abuse and mental illness at the same time. Loved ones can play a collaborative role here by engaging in a frank discussion of not only the genetics that might play a role in the newly sober person's emotional issues but also—to the extent that the newly sober is willing—the experiences that may have contributed to both problems. Naturally, a loved one is not a therapist—nor should he or she try to be. On the other hand, listening sympathetically and offering support have powerful healing effects in and of themselves.

Another important thing to keep in mind is how much getting sober can affect one's mental health. Sadly, many people get into substance use in an effort to control or heal their emotional problems only to have that use boomerang on them. They should know that research has supported the idea that getting sober in and of itself can help (although the best combination remains getting sober plus seeking professional help). Let's look at a couple of relevant research studies that shed light on the power of sobriety to heal.

In one study conducted by the VA healthcare system, 209 individuals who were diagnosed with both chronic depression and a severe alcohol-use disorder were recruited.[8] They were then randomly assigned to one of two treatments: cognitive-behavioral treatment (CBT) that was aimed at both the alcohol abuse and the depression but that did not advocate AA; and a treatment called Twelve-Step facilitation (TSF), which is aimed solely at treating substance abuse and which strongly encourages AA attendance and participation. All of the individuals of the study also received medication for their depression.

The researchers predicted that CBT would be superior to TSF on the basis that it was specifically designed to address both depression and substance abuse using cognitive-behavioral interventions whereas TSF's single goal was 12 Step fellowship involvement as a means of facilitating recovery. They measured depression and monitored both "drinking days" and "drinks per drinking day."

Here is a summary of their findings:

- Greater 12 Step meeting attendance and greater 12 Step fellowship involvement predicted both lower depression and less substance use.
- TSF led to significantly lower levels of depression during active treatment as compared to CBT.
- The positive effect of TSF on depression came directly as a result of meeting attendance, accounting for nearly one quarter of that effect.
- Lower depression scores at the three- and six-month follow-ups predicted lower drinking at months six and nine. That is, less drinking was associated with less depression.

This study ends with the following conclusion.

For patients with substance dependence and major depressive disorder, attendance at 12 step meetings is associated with mental health benefits that extend beyond substance use, and reduced depression could be a key mechanism whereby 12 step meetings reduce future drinking in this population.

Again, the position taken here is that the best course of action for someone who suffers from co-occurring substance abuse and a mental illness such as depression is to pursue both recovery and mental health treatment simultaneously. At the same time, it's important for both the newly sober and his or her loved ones to recognize the healing power of sobriety in and of itself.

A second population of individuals with co-occurring mental illness that has been the subject of research are those who suffer from PTSD. This study was spearheaded by Dr. Elisa Triffleman, who at the time of the research was affiliated with the department of psychiatry at Yale University School of Medicine. Her study, which compared two different approaches to treating PTSD, was reported in the journal *Alcoholism Treatment Quarterly*.[9]

The participants in this study were nine men and ten women who had been diagnosed with both PTSD and substance dependence (severe substance-use disorders involving alcohol or drugs). They were then randomly assigned to one of two treatments: substance dependency post-traumatic-stress-disorder therapy (SDPT) or TSF.

SDPT was a treatment that Dr. Triffleman and her coinvestigators devised and then predicted would be the more successful of the two treatments tested. SDPT, similar to the CBT model discussed above, was CBT that included components such as stress inoculation therapy, systematic desensitization, and in vivo exposure therapy. Systematic desensitization seeks to teach the client with PTSD first to relax and then to imagine a stressful event that is related to his or her PTSD, the idea being that this will help reduce symptoms such as anxiety. All of these strategies were incorporated in a single therapeutic package. Men and women assigned to the SDPT group completed an average of twenty-six individual therapy sessions.

TSF, as previously discussed, aims to facilitate active involvement in a 12 Step fellowship.[10] According to the researchers, TSF in this study was intended to serve as a control treatment. In other words, it was a treatment that was not expected to yield good results as compared to SDPT.

The men and women who were assigned to the TSF group completed an average of sixteen individual therapy sessions. The authors stated that the central hypotheses for this research were that

- treatment with SDPT would result in large decreases in substance-abuse severity as compared to treatment with TSF, and

- treatment with SDPT would lead to substantial decreases in PTSD symptoms and severity, and improvement on measures of overall mental health as compared to treatment with TSF.

It did not turn out that way. Here are the results as reported: "Other than for the SDPT participants receiving more therapy sessions than the TSF participants there were no significant differences in outcomes between treatments. In the sample as a whole there was improvement on measures of substance abuse, PTSD severity, and psychiatric severity."

What is most striking about these results is not that SDPT and TSF both worked but that once again a treatment that is aimed at 12 Step fellowship involvement would work as well for symptoms of PTSD as a treatment that was designed specifically to do so. The implication is clear: active involvement and commitment to a supportive fellowship like AA or the others we've reviewed appears to have healing powers beyond recovery from substance-use disorders alone.

THE VOYAGE MOVING FORWARD

Here are the lessons from the material in this chapter:

- A significant number of men and women are dealing with both a substance-use disorder and mental illness or emotional problems.
- It appears that substance abuse does not cause mental illness or emotional problems but rather that people are prone to using alcohol or drugs to self-medicate their emotional problems.
- The course of action with the best possible outcome is to pursue recovery from substance abuse and mental illness simultaneously.
- Although a combination of abstinence, counseling, and possibly medication is the recommended course of action, sobriety itself has been found to have a healing effect on emotional problems.

The newly sober individual and his or her loved ones need to embrace these findings and move forward collaboratively in following them.

· 9 ·

Healing Damaged Relationships

*C*arlier we covered the issue of how substance abuse, as it progresses along the substance-use spectrum, progressively "collapses" the user's lifestyle. Friends, work, favored activities, and so on gradually fade away as the relationship between the user and the substance advances from one that could be characterized as a casual acquaintance (low-risk use) to a commitment that, at its most extreme, takes precedence over all other commitments. Recovery, as we've seen, is in part a matter of recovering a lost lifestyle.

However, it is not only a lifestyle (people, places, routines, etc.) that must be rebuilt in recovery but also lost or damaged relationships. Researchers of child development have long recognized the problem that is created when a parent is separated from his or her child or children for a prolonged period of time—for example, due to serious illness resulting in a long hospitalization or institutionalization. When the parent returns home, they are often met not with the excitement or joy they might have hoped for but rather with indifference on the part of their children. It seems that deterioration of the parent-child relationship has a negative effect on attachment that in turn leads to alienation. It can take a long time to rebuild that attachment—if it can be rebuilt at all.

This chapter examines how a parallel process often takes place when a parent or partner is progressively lost to addiction. Psychologically, addiction is associated with "regression." In simple terms, as substance abuse progresses, the substance abuser progressively becomes less mature. If they are willing to reflect on this idea—and have the courage to face it—the newly sober man or woman can always relate to it. As uncomfortable as it may be, recognizing this process of regression can be the key to healing relationships that have been severely damaged as a result of substance abuse and addiction.

Bill Wilson, cofounder of AA, recognized this process in himself. He had established relationships with Carl Jung, a noted psychoanalyst, as well as Harry Tiebout, a psychiatrist in the United States. It was Tiebout who labeled the regression for Wilson, telling him that alcoholism had resulted in his becoming "his majesty the baby."[1] Not a particularly flattering characterization! Yet if we let ourselves get past that, it is possible to understand what is true about it. No matter how mature a substance abuser may have been at the outset, as substance use comes to play a greater and greater part in his or her life, the more childlike he or she will become—to the point where he or she may act in ways that are downright infantile.

Claire placed a call to a psychologist who she was told specialized in treating individuals with substance-abuse disorders. She was worried about her husband Everett. They'd been married twenty years and had two children, a son who'd recently gone off to a rather expensive private college and a daughter, Patrice, who was a junior in high school and contemplating a similar path forward. Everett had always liked his cocktails and wine, Claire explained, but over the past year his drinking had become worse. With degrees in engineering and business, he was a successful executive with a firm that did business not only within the United States but overseas as well. This required some travel on Everett's part.

It seemed to Claire that Everett's drinking had increased along with stress at work. The company was facing increased international competition, and as vice president for foreign sales, Everett was involved in developing products—at times collaboratively with foreign firms—that could compete in an increasingly intense and competitive business environment. This meant careful attention not only to design details but to efficient manufacturing and effective communication as well. To add to the picture, Claire had discovered that Everett, on one of his overseas trips, had learned that he could obtain tranquilizers without a prescription in one of the countries he visited. He'd started using these on occasion as a way of coping with job pressures and helping him fall asleep, in addition to drinking, but over time he had come to stashing quantities in his luggage and around the house, which Claire discovered while searching a cabinet for a light bulb. When she asked

Everett about it, he admitted that he was now using the tranquilizers on pretty much a daily basis, but he argued that they helped.

Between the tranquilizers and the liquor, Claire explained, Everett had gradually retreated even more from family life than his job had required before. Their daughter was keenly aware of this and had even remarked sarcastically about it on a few occasions. Everett had snapped back, accusing his daughter of being "a spoiled brat." And when Claire brought it up his reaction was similar: She didn't appreciate all he did for her and the family, he said, adding that he was fine and she should leave him alone.

At that point Everett had stopped going to the gym he used to use twice a week, where he'd meet with two longstanding male friends and go for a beer afterward. He now typically retired to bed much earlier than in the past, often foregoing the nightly news that he and Claire had watched together for many years. Once, when Patrice called Everett to ask if he could meet her for the kind of occasional father-daughter dinner they'd once enjoyed, and added that she'd prefer he not drink beforehand, he threw what she described as a tantrum, yelled at her, and hung up on her.

Everett had become increasingly irritable and impatient and would "go off" at the least frustration. "He wants what he wants, and he wants it now," Claire explained. Being around him had become so difficult that she'd taken to minimizing daily contact with him. In addition, based on some comments he'd made, Claire was worried that Everett's job might actually be in jeopardy as a result of declining performance on his part.

Everett is a good example of this process of regression that goes along with worsening substance abuse. In order to rise to where he was in the business world, he had to be intelligent, but he also had to learn to be patient, to learn at times to delay short-term gratification (an immediate sale at a bad price) in the interest of long-term gains. His position also demanded good interpersonal communication skills and a capacity for collaboration. As he progressively fell victim to mild, moderate, and eventually severe substance abuse, however, these personal qualities deteriorated to the point where he really did act like a small child whose world centered around him and who "wanted what he wanted and when he wanted it." He had little tolerance for frustration and (as when he hung up the phone on his daughter) would easily throw a tantrum. This is, of course, normal for a young child, as every parent can attest. But as we mature, we gradually grow out of this developmental stage. Addiction reverses this process. Accordingly, recovery requires that both the newly sober man or woman and his or her loved ones acknowledge this and determine to change it.

SUBSTANCE ABUSE AND DAMAGED ATTACHMENTS

As the example of Everett shows, the person with a severe substance-use disorder was not necessarily born immature; rather, it is the addictive process itself that causes this regression. In a way parallel to the way that prolonged parental absence leads to a gradual deterioration of the parent-child attachment (leading to an indifference or alienation that becomes evident when the parent returns home), so addiction creates alienation and broken attachments. That was the case for Everett, Claire, and his children. As it turned out, Patrice's brother, Ned, felt pretty much the same as she did: increasingly detached from Everett. That was why he said that he was planning to remain at college and take summer classes rather than return home. Everett sensed all of this alienation, but he did not take responsibility for it. At the time of this writing, he has still not accepted his substance-abuse problem or sought help for it. He stands the risk of never beginning a voyage to recovery but rather becoming shipwrecked and sinking.

Maria is another example. Having become dependent on prescription painkillers combined with daily tranquilizer use over a period of four years, like Everett she had retreated more and more from family life. A real estate agent in a large city, Maria was financially successful. Between her income and that of her husband, Matthew, they could afford a comfortable lifestyle for themselves and their three children. She was fortunate in that she could pretty much schedule her own working hours and was able to work from home, spending little time in the realty office.

Maria was what is sometimes referred to as a "high-functioning addict" in that she was able, on one level, to continue her job and avoid failure on that level. At home, however, it was a different matter. Although Matthew and her teenage daughters understood that Maria suffered from chronic pain due to severe arthritis, they also knew from experience that as time went on, she could be counted on less and less as a functioning member of the family. Her daily routine included taking a painkiller first thing when she woke up and then taking a tranquilizer first thing when she got home from showing a home or condo. All in all she interacted less and less with Matthew and the girls, who collectively had taken over responsibility for preparing meals, cleaning up, doing laundry, and so on. And while they understood her issues, they also all found themselves more or less going their separate ways while Maria retreated to her bedroom typically by eight, took another tranquilizer (and maybe an extra painkiller as well), and fell asleep.

In significant ways, Maria's addiction separated her from her family just as prolonged hospitalization can damage the parent-child attachment. Things began to fall apart for her, however, when she took a tranquilizer and pain pill together after leaving a home showing and rear-ended another car when she failed to hit her brakes in time at a stoplight. The officer who responded to the scene couldn't help but notice that Maria looked impaired, and though she denied drinking he insisted on bringing her to an emergency room for an assessment. It was then her substance abuse came to light. Not only Matthew but also the two doctors Maria had been getting these medications from for a long time were notified by the emergency room physician, who advised the doctors to reconsider their prescribing practices while also insisting that Maria make an appointment on the spot at the hospital's addiction services treatment division. She spent the night at the hospital while receiving replacement medication intended to prevent withdrawal symptoms, and she went to the treatment center the next day.

Recovering from her dependency on pain medication as well as tranquilizers was not easy for Maria. Just as her family had been hesitant to confront the reality of her addiction for what it was, so had she. When it finally became obvious, after the accident, she agreed to start treatment. This included medication to temporarily replace the prescription pain medication that she was truly dependent upon plus tapering off the tranquilizers. Through counseling she was guided into making many of the lifestyle changes discussed here, starting with learning to practice mindfulness meditation,[2] a technique that research has found to be effective in managing pain; adding physical therapy aimed at helping her arthritis; and changing her diet. Her family stood firmly behind her in these efforts.

After a difficult first month, Maria was beginning, in her words, to feel "like the human being I used to be." That was all well and good. However, as she began to recover her past self, Maria got a sense that her relationship with her husband and her daughters was not really very good. They supported her, to be sure, but she did not feel very connected to any of them and sensed that there was distance between them. Her counselor explained that this was to be expected and that they should work together on it.

LEARNING TO LISTEN

One more example is Hannah. The wife of a very successful business-man, she had never had to work but rather occupied herself with various charities as well as a good deal of socializing with other women in similar circumstances. During their youngest years her two daughters and son had known Hannah as an attentive mother who gave them attention and brought them to the various activities they signed up for. But after her father died in a plane crash, Hannah started drinking. Over time her drinking increased, and her involvement with the children (as well as with her husband) gradually decreased to the point where when the kids were in their twenties, they mutually acknowledged that Hannah was an alcoholic and chose to spend less and less time around her. Hannah did not see the connection between this increasing alienation and her drinking but attributed it instead to the children just getting older. However, after she experienced two blackouts on two different holidays, her husband and children organized an intervention, confronted Hannah about her drinking, and demanded that she go for treatment.

Hannah did go for treatment, where she admitted that she had a drinking problem, but then she left treatment early, determined to stop drinking. She went to AA and did stop drinking. However, what she still did not do was connect the dots between her longstanding alcoholism and the alienation that had developed in her relationship with her children. In communications among themselves they shared that they were glad that Hannah had stopped drinking, but her daughters in particular expressed frustration that they had never been able to talk with their mother about how much her alcoholism had robbed them of a close relationship with her over the years. They decided they needed to talk with her about that and arranged to meet her at the family house, ostensibly for lunch but in reality to share their feelings.

The meeting did not go well. It began with Hannah basically talking about how well her sobriety was going. She was attending three AA meetings a week, she said, and had a sponsor she really liked. She claimed she had no desire to drink. The girls congratulated her on those achievements, but then the older one said that she wanted to share some uncomfortable feelings and began to express both sadness and some anger over the fact that alcoholism had robbed her and her siblings of a relationship with Hannah for many years.

Hannah's reaction was not good. She got defensive. Her response to her daughters went something like this: "If my drinking made you uncomfortable, I'm sorry. But I'm sober now, and it's time for all of us to move on." This kind of response avoids accepting the reality of how substance abuse can severely damage close relationships and how the substance abuser's relationship with alcohol or drugs comes over time to displace his or her relationships with loved ones. On the one hand, if they complain about this, they may experience the kind of regressive reaction that Everett gave to his daughter. On the other hand, if they avoid such confrontations, they may be left to simply become gradually less attached to and more alienated from the substance abuser, which is what happened between Hannah and her children.

Relationships between a newly sober person and his or her loved ones not likely to heal unless the newly sober individual is able to connect the dots and accept the reality that their growing relationship with alcohol or drugs has gradually replaced their former relationships —with children, with partners, with friends, and with other family. A failure to do so, moreover, will only prolong alienation and pose a risk to recovery. As much as Hannah's children wanted to support her sobriety, for example, her refusal to accept how her addiction had affected these relationships stood as a barrier to the emotional connections that could support it. Hannah's connection to AA was important, to be sure, but a true connection to others is equally desirable.

In Maria's case the outcome was better. Unlike Hannah, she was able to recognize, with the help of her counselor, how her addiction to painkillers and tranquilizers had gradually resulted in her becoming an absentee family member. When the counselor suggested they schedule a couple of family sessions to address this, Maria agreed. These sessions were not easy. Maria did, however, make it clear from the outset that she took responsibility for how her addiction had affected the family and that she wanted to hear about it. Those sessions, in turn, marked a change in the family dynamics. Maria's openness allowed the family members to first express their sadness and anger over having lost her to addiction and then to begin the process of rebuilding those relationships. In terms of Maria's voyage to recovery, these healed relationships would prove to be an important source of support.

ESTABLISHING SHARED GOALS

For many loved ones of newly sober individuals, the process of establishing honest communication as described above is critical to a collaborative recovery. This makes sense as it's easy to understand how a partner or child could remain alienated if the pain they endured as a consequence of addiction is not at least acknowledged. There may be little more that the newly sober person can do other than to be open to hearing this without dismissing or minimizing it. Most people are quite receptive to that kind of acknowledgment. If the newly sober man or woman and his or her loved ones have not engaged in that kind of dialogue yet, it is time to do so now.

Perhaps nothing contributes to cohesiveness in relationships and family life more than shared values and goals. The most cohesive families are bound by a shared commitment to a way of life and to goals that motivate them. Some of these may seem rather simple: preparing meals, maintaining a house (including cleaning and repairs), and perhaps doing yardwork or schoolwork. If children are involved, commitments to their schooling, health care, and activities can also be a part of these shared commitments. For some families, religious activities constitute yet another common bond. Then there may be broader goals: financing a child's college education, saving for a better home, and so on.

The process of regression that comes as substance abuse progresses along the substance-use spectrum involves the steady erosion of the individual's lifestyle so that it comes over time to revolve more and more around the singular goal of getting and staying intoxicated or high. This leads to a shrinking not only of the substance abuser's lifestyle but also impacts the lifestyles that once characterized his or her primary relationship and family. The typical process is that addiction leads those who are in close relationships with the substance abuser to progressively pursue separate agendas as the agenda for the substance abuser comes to revolve increasingly around substance use. In time their goals and priorities may diverge so much that they have little in the way of common interests or priorities. On returning from rehab or being discharged from treatment, the now sober partner or parent may find it a challenge to accept the reality that his or her children or spouse have in fact actually developed lifestyles apart from his or her decidedly limited one. A stark choice then becomes clear: to continue to pursue separate lifestyles or seek to work together to establish some degree of common ground that can help bind their relationships and family together and support recovery.

If partners, or the family as a whole, choose the second option, they first need to openly acknowledge the drifting apart that may have occurred as a result of substance abuse. Partners and children, for example, may have developed relationships that have largely or completely excluded the substance abuser. It's common, for example, for children to report that they rarely if ever invite friends to their house because a parent's substance abuse is common knowledge and an embarrassment. Similarly, spouses may have cultivated new friends. Activities that now play an important role in the lives of family members may be foreign to the newly sober individual. More than one teen has reported that a parent never attended one of their high school games, inquired about their experiences at school, or went with them to see a movie. Reports like these clearly attest to the separate lifestyles that substance abuse can create. For all of these reasons, a dialogue about how separate lifestyles have evolved and now exist is an almost mandatory starting point. What follows are some guidelines for ways to reverse this process and begin to build a shared lifestyle.

Don't Expect Everyone to Be Equally on Board

It isn't reasonable to expect other family members to abruptly abandon whatever separate lifestyles they've developed just because the former substance abuser enters rehab or treatment and gets sober. Children are not going to simply give up friends the substance abuser does not know or activities that involve those friends. Spouses should not be asked to abandon friends they may have made to compensate for a deteriorated marital relationship. To some extent the newly sober person needs to come to terms with these changes—without falling victim to either resentment or excessive guilt—and accept them as part of a new, sober reality.

Gradually Develop New Aspects of Existing Relationships

Taking the examples given above, a newly sober parent of teens can begin by asking if it would be okay for him or her to attend a sport that their child is involved in or to perhaps see a movie together that both would like to see. Taking a child out for a quick breakfast or lunch is another good option. These things do not ask the child to give up whatever social network they may have developed. On the contrary, the newly sober parent needs to accept the fact that this may only change slowly, if ever. Meanwhile, these kinds of shared activities can help to rebuild a parent-child relationship that has fallen victim to alienation.

The same idea applies to partners who may have developed relationships with friends outside the marriage. As opposed to trying to insert himself or herself into these relationships, a better approach for the newly sober individual would be to accept them while beginning to rebuild the marital relationship. Identify common interests and pursue them. As with children, keep shared activities comfortable; as suggested above, breakfast or lunch is a great start.

Open Communication around New Family Rituals

We previously discussed how rituals can support substance abuse and how an active substance abuser establishes such rituals, often replacing prior ones. Examples include the man who retreats to his basement workshop immediately on getting home from work and drinks or lights up a cannabis smoke. Or the woman who ritually drinks glass after glass of wine while preparing dinner and catching the news on TV. Rituals can extend to favorite clothing, favorite music, and even favorite glasses for drinking wine, beer, or whiskey. One woman purchased a case of six identical wine glasses in case she accidentally broke one!

Families also tend to develop and follow certain rituals over time. Weekly religious services and Sunday dinner are examples, though others include attending children's athletic events, shopping, cooking, playing games, or watching particular television shows together. As one family member gradually succumbs to addiction, however, these rituals are usually disrupted. The Sunday family dinner may fade away, and it may be only one parent (or a grandparent) who occasionally attends a game. Part of building a robust recovery means changing routines by abandoning those that supported substance abuse and substituting ones that do two things: support recovery and build family cohesiveness. Here is an example.

Ned and his brother Chris inherited their father's small construction company and grew it over a decade into a large firm that specialized in building custom homes as well as medium-size buildings for companies. Both brothers tended to devote long hours to the business, but while Chris also spent considerable time interacting with his wife and children, Ned had slipped over time into the daily drinking pattern that had been his father's lifestyle. As a result, as compared to Chris, Ned had become pretty much an absentee father and husband. One of his sons was an avid swimmer who was captain of his high school swim team while his other son was more academically and community inclined, excelling in school and becoming president of the school's student council. However, Ned was not really privy to or part of any of these things. Instead, he would pour himself a large glass of bourbon after work, plant himself in a favored lounger, and watch his favored television shows. On the few occasions that his wife complained about this routine, Ned responded with defensiveness and anger. He had a demanding and stressful job, he said, and that was his way of relaxing. "I deserve it," he said, "because I work all day to support this family."

As you might expect, Ned's family life was nothing to speak of. The kind of alienation and drifting apart that we've discussed typified Ned's day-to-day life. Though Ned's wife cooked dinner daily, family members rarely ate together. Instead, the boys would fill their plates and retreat to their bedrooms where they would eat, do homework, and either play computer games or talk with friends through their phones or via social media. They never invited friends to the house. They did not talk to Ned about their outside activities or share their respective successes other than with their mother now and then. Ned's wife, meanwhile, had become active in their church and was on several committees there. It was, in a word, a family whose members existed in isolation from one another and led essentially parallel lives.

The consequences that led Ned to face his alcoholism are ones we are already familiar with, and they had to do with his health: he suffered a heart attack while at work and ended up hospitalized, where he learned that he had hypertension and a fatty liver and that he needed to have three stents inserted in a cardiac artery. His doctors also frankly confronted Ned about his drinking and told him that if he did not quit, his prognosis for a long life was decidedly limited. If he could not quit by himself, they strongly recommended reaching out for help.

A week after he returned home from the hospital, Ned's wife discovered two bottles of bourbon stashed in different places around the house. This time when she confronted Ned, it amounted to an ultimatum: either he get help to stop drinking or move out. Their sons were completely aware of his situation, she said, and she felt that Ned just going along as usual was an unacceptable model for them.

Ned did get sober. Though he tried both SMART Recovery and AA (hating them both at first), he complied with a condition of the agency where he was getting treatment and agreed to attend one AA meeting per week. His counselor guided him in trying out different meetings, and after four months of sobriety he did find one—as well as one other man—that he actually felt comfortable with. That marked the point of departure for Ned's voyage to recovery.

It took nearly a year—with the help of his counselor along with an AA sponsor—for Ned to come to terms with just how much his alcohol abuse had distorted both his own and his family's life. His first step in repairing that damage was to ask for a family meeting (something Ned had never done), where he steeled himself and (being sober for the first time in as long as he could recall) owned up to this and apologized. He said he did not expect applause for this admission but rather that he hoped that together the family could begin the process of rebuilding. At his counselor's suggestion, he said that he would like to try establishing some small but important new rituals and routines among them, and he then opened the meeting to suggestions. His wife piped up first, saying that one thing she really missed were the Sunday family dinners, which she said they'd enjoyed when the boys were very young but that had faded away into nothing more than Thanksgiving dinner.

Ned's sons both said they wanted to think about it, though both told Ned that they did appreciate what he'd done with the family meeting. Two days later his younger son—the academic one—said that one thing he enjoyed doing was visiting a local flea market on occasion but that he'd always gone either alone or with a friend. He asked Ned if that would be something he'd like to do, and Ned jumped at the chance. The following week Ned asked his other son if it would be okay if he came to watch the boy's swim meets and got another okay.

These changes might seem minimal, but they marked a significant change in Ned's lifestyle as well as in his role within the family. His counselor and sponsor praised Ned both for his courage to face up to the effects of his addiction on the family as well as his openness to these changes. His counselor shared his belief that these marked just the beginning of what he was certain would mark further changes that would build family cohesiveness and support Ned's recovery.

This chapter extends the boundaries and the very definition of recovery. By now it should be clear that recovery extends well beyond treatment or rehab and is much broader in scope. Hopefully it is also clear that a robust and resilient recovery is best approached as a collaborative, as opposed to solo, endeavor, bringing the newly sober person and his or her loved ones together as joint stakeholders in recovery.

· 10 ·

Spirituality and Recovery

$\mathcal{W}$hen I first began to speak on this topic—the role that spirituality can play in recovery—I was greeted with a lot of skepticism. Colleagues and therapists expressed opinions like "Spirituality is too vague a concept to be studied" or "I don't think that therapists should be telling clients what they should believe" or "I don't see a connection between spirituality and sobriety."

Over time, two responses to such criticisms have evolved in my thinking. First, it turns out that researchers have indeed developed ways of studying spirituality and its role in recovery from substance abuse. Second, people—in particular skeptics—often tend to equate spirituality with religion, but the truth is that they are different. To be sure virtually all religions advocate spirituality, but one can live a spiritual lifestyle without being a member of any formal religion.

DEFINING SPIRITUALITY

Although people sometimes equate spirituality with religious practice, it is possible to define spirituality independent of religiosity. One way to think of spirituality is to recognize that it consists of the values and priorities we hold along with how closely our day-to-day lives are consistent with those values and priorities. This is in fact how researchers have gone about defining and studying spirituality. More about that soon.

SPIRITUALITY AND SUBSTANCE ABUSE

Virtually all of the individuals whose stories have been told in this book so far can attest to how substance abuse led to a steady deterioration in any spirituality they once had. They will tell you that as their substance abuse worsened along the spectrum, they increasingly acted in ways that betrayed whatever values and priorities they once had. They became dishonest and deceitful, groomed enablers to feed their habit, and neglected responsibilities and their commitments to relationships. They became self-absorbed. And so on. In this way substance abuse is a pathway to shame. On some level the substance abuser is aware of how substance abuse came to overtake whatever they once valued or admired in others and what they once wished to embrace in their own lives. Heroes fall by the wayside and are replaced by cynicism. Shame can be a powerful (and negative) motivator. It may be the one emotion that the newly sober man or woman wishes most to deny. Yet left to fester, it can easily sabotage recovery.

WHAT WE KNOW ABOUT
SPIRITUALITY AND RECOVERY

Over the past decade or more, qualified researchers at academic institutions have taken on the challenge of examining how spirituality might play a role in supporting recovery. It's important that we understand what this research tells us, as it can be a guide for the newly sober and his or her loved ones as well on to how to reverse the process of spiritual deterioration. The first study we'll look at was conducted by Stephanie Carroll of the California School of Professional Psychology.[1] Dr. Carroll recruited a sample of one hundred AA members (fifty-one male) from twenty different AA groups in northern California. Her goal was to evaluate the relationship between these men's and women's spiritual practices and their recovery. To do this, of course, she needed first to define spirituality in some way and then measure it.

Dr. Carroll decided to define spirituality in terms of Steps 11 and 12 of the AA program. Step 11 recommends the practice of meditation or prayer, and Step 12 has to do with altruism—especially reaching out to the newly sober. While these are not aspects of any specific religion, most would agree that these activities meet the criteria for being manifestations of what we commonly think of as spirituality.

Step 11 and 12 activities were measured using a questionnaire that Dr. Carroll devised. It asked respondents to indicate how often they engaged in each of a number of activities, from daily to yearly. Here are some of the activities that the questionnaire asked about:

- prayer
- meditation
- reading spiritual material (for example, daily meditations)
- spending time in nature (for example, hiking or camping)
- interacting with art (for example, visiting a museum or painting or drawing)
- attending a religious service
- greeting a newcomer at an AA meeting
- engaging in AA service activities
- engaging in non–AA community service activities
- volunteering to be an AA sponsor or temporary sponsor

In this sample of active AA members, more than half reported praying or meditating twice a day as well as reading some form of spiritual literature three times a week. Half also reported listening to music that they defined as spiritual—meaning that it was music that was consistent with meditation or prayer—on a weekly basis. Half also said that they interacted with art in some way at least monthly. Interestingly, despite these spiritual activities, less than one-half of the sample reported attending formal religious services. On the other hand, 90 percent said they attended AA meetings at least twice a week. It would seem, then, that it was AA rather than an organized religion that was the driving force behind these spiritual activities (not that this suggests that individuals should not attend religious services if they so choose).

Dr. Carroll's questionnaire also asked respondents to indicate their current length of sobriety in years and months. She then compared this to how the men and women in her sample scored on her spirituality scale.

What Dr. Carroll found was that those activities most closely associated with Step 11, such as meditation, prayer, reading spiritual literature, and activities such as connecting with art or nature were significantly correlated with length of sobriety. In other words, engaging in these spiritual activities was associated with a more robust recovery. Attending AA meetings was associated with better recovery; but the spiritual activities in and of themselves were independently predictive of longer recovery.

In a second study, a group of researchers headed by Dr. John Kelly of the Department of Psychiatry at Massachusetts General Hospital and Harvard Medical School also decided to venture into this concept of spirituality and what role it might play in recovery.[2] Using a large sample of 1,726 men and women who had undergone treatment for alcohol-use disorders, the researchers looked at three variables:

- alcohol use—The researchers used measures of percent days abstinent (PDA) and drinks per drinking day (DDD), which are pretty much standard measures in substance-abuse research. PDA indicates the extent to which an individual abstains totally from alcohol while DDD measures how many drinks a person consumes on a day when they "slip."
- AA attendance—This was a simple measure: how many AA meetings an individual attended in the previous ninety days.
- spirituality—To gauge spirituality these researchers employed a measure called the Religious Background and Behavior (RBB) questionnaire. The RBB is worth a closer look to see exactly how its authors define spirituality.

The RBB was developed by Gerard Connors of the Research Institute on Addictions and J. Scott Tonigan and William R. Miller of the University of New Mexico.[3] They utilized a combination of self-identification along with an inventory of specific activities and experiences to capture and quantify the extent to which spirituality plays a role in an individual's life. For example, the person taking the RBB is first asked to identify him or herself as

- atheist: doesn't believe in God
- agnostic: believes we can't really know about God
- unsure: doesn't know what to believe about God

- spiritual: believes in God but is not religious
- religious: believes in God and practices a religion

Next, the individual taking the RBB is asked to estimate how often they engage in different activities on an eight-point scale that ranges from "Never" to "More than once a day." They include activities such as

- praying
- meditating
- attending religious services
- reading holy or spiritual writings

If you recall, in her study of spirituality and recovery, Stephanie Carroll found that the recovering men and women showed a significant increase in spiritual beliefs that was correlated with AA involvement, yet less than half of them attended formal religious services. In their study, Kelly and colleagues found that higher scores on the spirituality-religiousness scale were positively related to PDA (abstinence) and negatively related to DDD (drinking). In other words, men and women who reported stronger spiritual beliefs were indeed more likely to remain abstinent and also to drink less if they did slip.

In addition to the above, these researchers found that spirituality-religiousness increased as their subjects attended more AA meetings over time. This too suggests that it is active involvement in AA over time that has the effect of promoting spiritual beliefs. The authors conclude,

> Results from this study, using a large multi-site clinical sample, exhibiting a broad range of alcohol-related involvement and impairment, support the central idea espoused by AA that spirituality is important in recovery and that AA appears to mobilize spiritual changes, which help explain AA's beneficial effects on recovery from alcohol dependence.

Despite the fact that many people hold the view that spirituality is too vague a concept to quantify and study scientifically, it's apparent that we can draw several conclusions from the above research. The first is that because AA emphasizes spirituality, those who identify with

AA and follow its program by and large do become more spiritual over time. That said, it is also the case that other recovery fellowships (such as Women for Sobriety) that advocate for spiritual values such as altruism, humility, and faith in the collective power of fellowship can also promote spiritual development. Second, we can say with certitude that spiritual growth itself appears to contribute in a positive way to sustained recovery.

MOVING TOWARD A SPIRITUAL LIFESTYLE

Understandably, a substance abuser who is newly sober may be defensive when it comes to looking back on how substance abuse progressively eroded his or her capacity for living up to values and priorities that he or she once held dear. However, as uncomfortable as it may be, men and women who are in sustained recovery attest to just how healing such a personal inventory can be and how embracing spiritual values as represented by fellowships such as AA and Women for Sobriety freed them to move forward with their recovery.

Jane worked as an office manager for a dentist who was also a longstanding friend of the family. She was competent in her work, but at some point her boyfriend introduced her to cocaine. Her substance abuse did not progress to the point where she needed rehab, but it got bad enough that she started stealing small amounts of money from the practice to buy cocaine. Since she was the one responsible for maintaining the books, she found it relatively easy to "skim" money on a weekly basis. And since she also prepared the taxes, she found that she could understate the practice income so as to cover her tracks.

In addition to stealing from the dental practice, Jane stole from her mother. Jane managed her aging mother's finances. Her mother never questioned Jane but assumed that she was always acting responsibly. Yet here too, Jane eventually took to skimming money for cocaine.

After about a year, Jane's relationship with her boyfriend dissolved in large part because he not only used cocaine but was pressing Jane to steal more and more to feed his as well as her habit. She decided to confide her habit to her doctor, who prescribed something to ease the discomfort that she was sure Jane would experience should she quit.

The doctor advocated quitting, of course, and offered to refer Jane to a treatment center if needed.

Jane did indeed experience discomfort when she quit cocaine. The medication helped. She took a few days off from work with the excuse of having caught a virus. By the time three weeks had passed she was in her own words "beginning to feel like Jane again." Looking back, she described the past year of her life as surreal. She wasn't sure exactly why she'd been persuaded to try cocaine other than that her boyfriend had been very attractive and at least initially paid a lot of attention to her. Before meeting him, she said, she would have described herself as pretty much a "straight arrow." She'd done well in school, never getting into trouble. Right through college she'd attended religious services fairly regularly. And she'd had good friends—at least until she got into the cocaine. As that got worse, she let those friendships drift away, making excuses for not getting together until people stopped asking. When one close friend asked Jane if she was okay, Jane offered the weak excuse that between work, her mother, and her boyfriend she had little time for anything else. She didn't believe her friend found that explanation convincing, but the friend didn't press the issue.

As much as Jane felt physically better over time, what she'd done while being caught in the throes of a growing addiction hung over her like a cloud. She felt terribly guilty about stealing money from her employer and mother, and she also felt guilty about more or less abandoning her friends. In a follow-up with her doctor she shared some of this, and the doctor told Jane she should probably talk to a counselor—one who was experienced in helping people with substance-abuse issues. It was through that counseling that Jane was able to take stock, make reparations, and move forward in recovery.

Jane asked for a meeting with the dentist, where she confessed to having skimmed as much as a few thousand dollars from the practice. She admitted to the cocaine use, told the dentist that she had stopped and was working with both her own doctor and a therapist, and that it was her intention to gradually replace what she had taken, though it would take about a year. She and her therapist agreed that it would probably hurt Jane's mother too much if Jane were to tell her about stealing money. Instead, Jane made a similar determination to replace what she'd taken, again over time. As for her friends, Jane confided that she'd gotten into cocaine with the boyfriend but that she had stopped and hoped to rekindle those friendships.

Jane is a good example of a person who had the courage to confront the ways in which substance abuse had compromised her integrity and led her to do things she would never have thought herself capable of. The shame she experienced could, if allowed to fester, have constituted a threat to her continued sobriety. She did not allow that to happen. The reality is that most people are open to sincere apologies. Most people are capable of forgiveness especially if the apology is perceived as sincere and followed up by a perceived determination to do better. However, if the apology is perceived as merely placating, the response may not be so positive. The spouse abuser who expresses guilt and apologizes after beating his wife and who comes home with flowers may lack credibility if his spouse does not believe he is sincere and the abuse is likely to be repeated.

Consistent with the example provided by Jane, here are a few guidelines for the newly sober and their loved ones for approaching this issue of spirituality and incorporating it in a recovery plan.

Don't Deny Reality

The fact is that just as substance abuse results in regression as it progresses along the substance-use spectrum, so does it gradually lead to a spiritual erosion, assuming we define spirituality as the values and priorities we hold dear and wish to live by. Substance abusers, in other words, are not born immature or immoral; rather, substance abuse causes these personality changes. As painful and damaging as these changes may be—for relationships, for careers, for health, and so on—they are a reality that the substance abuser typically does not inflict intentionally on himself or herself or on his or her loved ones. Healing begins when the newly sober individual is able to do the following: first, accept, rather than deny or minimize, the ways in which substance abuse led them to act in ways that they would at one time not have condoned or approved of; and second, make a sincere apology and show a sincere desire to reverse this process moving forward.

Pursue Spiritual Activities

The research studies we reviewed were based on being able to come up with a definition of what it means to be spiritual and then determining how spirituality relates to staying clean and sober. That's about as good a guideline as we could hope for. We know from this research that spiritual practices support recovery and that those in recovery are inclined to increase spiritual activities over time. One question is, Can the newly sober as well as their loved ones take advantage of these findings? Is the pursuit of spirituality equally good for the newly sober and his or her loved ones? I would argue that it is. Accordingly, the newly sober person (along with his or her loved ones) should consider gradually adding one or more of the following to his or her lifestyle:

- meditation or prayer—Many daily meditation books are available and offer a good way of starting each day. Some have religious themes while others do not. Either way, they offer a good way of "grounding" at the start of each day.
- community service—Altruism is an important spiritual value, and a decision to participate in some form of community service, no matter how minor, can make a big difference in one's life.
- connecting with art or nature—Join a club that sponsors nature walks (or just take them yourself, better yet with a loved one). Visit an art museum now and then and spend some time contemplating what you see.
- listening to soothing music—Playing such music in the company of loved ones can help promote bonding and healing.
- attending religious services—If you believe that this should be a part of your life, or your family life, try to connect or reconnect with your chosen religion.

Clearly spirituality involves getting in touch with those values and priorities we value and that we would like to live by. Integrating activities consistent with these values and priorities can strengthen the kind of collaborative recovery advocated here.

What If It Doesn't Work?

Analyzing Slips and Relapses

$\mathcal{N}$aturally every newly sober person and his or her loved ones reading this book hopes that all of the guidelines described here will lead to a robust and resilient recovery—resilient in the sense that it leads to a sobriety that can stand up to stresses and strains. Recovery is not easily accomplished, however, as all of those who have experienced either temporary slips or major relapses know all too well. Even the best-laid plans can go awry, and even the best of intentions are not always sufficient to achieve a goal. With that in mind it's imperative that we move on to discussing the next best things to do if one of these events happen.

Slips, and even full relapses, should not be cause for despair but neither should they be quickly dismissed. A simple "I'm okay now" following a slip into drinking or drug use could set the stage for a lengthy relapse by falsely implying there's nothing to worry about. It may be tempting to seek solace in such an attitude, but it is dangerous thinking.

We begin by examining how a slip or relapse can be analyzed to inform the individual whose recovery has slipped, along with his or her loved ones, of what might need to change. In many cases this also means what might need to be avoided. There are three contexts, or dimensions, that define a slip or relapse: the cognitive context, the social context, and the emotional context. We will examine each of these and what they have to teach us. For purposes of discussion, we can think of a slip as a single or time-limited event in which the newly sober person drinks or uses former drugs of choice. In contrast, a relapse means a complete return to prior alcohol or drug use.

THE COGNITIVE CONTEXT

The cognitive context can be summed up this way: "What were you thinking at the time of your slip or relapse?" This brings us back to an important discussion we had earlier and that is what the newly treated individual truly believes about his or her substance abuse. We reviewed research on moderation and so-called controlled use as well as what difference a person's goal makes for their chances of recovery. We learned that men and women who choose abstinence over controlled use have the best outcomes and that research on moderation and controlled use shows poor results at best. Nevertheless, despite these realities, substance abusers and the general public are probably familiar with programs or techniques that promise success along with the idea that abstinence is not a necessary goal. These approaches have obvious appeal as they suggest (implicitly if not overtly) that "you don't have to give it up entirely" in order to mitigate the consequences of substance abuse and return to a normal lifestyle.

Earlier it was recommended that the individual newly discharged from rehab or treatment do an honest self-assessment of what he or she really believes about his or her substance abuse and whether he or she honestly believes that abstinence is the best goal to pursue. It was also recommended, because loved ones are also stakeholders in the recovery journey, that they and the newly sober person discuss this issue frankly. In response to a slip or relapse, it is time to repeat both parts of that exercise: both self-assessment and dialogue. The following questions can be a guide for both:

- What role, if any, did loved ones play in my initial decision to enter rehab or treatment? Was there an intervention in which I was faced with consequences if I did not agree to treatment?
- At the time I entered rehab or treatment, how would I have described my substance use? Was it mild? Moderate? Severe?
- Did I believe when I entered treatment that I really needed to abstain?
- On leaving rehab or treatment, was I holding on to any idea that I could control or moderate my use as opposed to abstaining?
- When I had my slip or relapse, what goal was I pursuing? Controlled use? Abstinence?

- What were the consequences of my slip or relapse? Do I believe it hurt my relationships with my loved ones? Do they believe it hurt these relationships?
- Finally, what is my thinking at this point about my goal with respect to alcohol or drug use moving forward?

As it turns out, the above cognitive context actually applies much more often to slips and relapses than many newly sober individuals are inclined to admit. Although they may have recognized that they had a serious problem when they agreed to enter rehab or treatment and may have publicly said so, privately they may have harbored the notion that they could somehow manage the problem without having to totally give up alcohol or drugs. Truth be told, that was exactly the attitude of the founders of AA prior to their establishing the first AA meeting—and it remains the hidden thinking of many men and women who need to experience progressively worse consequences before taking the cognitive leap of admitting that they need to abstain.

For others, the cognitive context of a slip can be different. One young man, Michael, was hospitalized following a party at his college during which he drank so much that he passed out and nearly choked on his own vomit. His fellow partiers dialed 911, and Michael was taken in an ambulance to the hospital.

It turned out that drinking this heavily was not an unusual event for this young man. On his arrival at the hospital, it was determined that his blood alcohol level was dangerously close to the poisonous level and that his life could be in danger. He then spent the next two days in the hospital, at which point his parents picked him up and drove him directly to a rehab facility. Michael spent the next two weeks there, attending group therapy sessions daily and AA meetings.

Michael's heavy drinking had started early in high school. He described himself as socially extremely anxious and insecure about his appearance and attractiveness as well as his intelligence. He attributed his ability to socialize to the fact that he would drink in anticipation of virtually any social activity. In an inebriated state, he found his anxiety decreased enough so that he was able to talk, joke, and get along with his peers—who generally didn't know he was drunk. Once at a party, he'd continue to drink. He was even able to flirt with women he found attractive though he'd never had a steady girlfriend.

In treatment Michael admitted that he had a drinking problem, that it was bad, and that it was dangerous. But when he attended the AA meetings and therapy groups in rehab, he sometimes had his doubts that he was "as bad as the others" in treatment or those who told their stories at AA meetings. After he was discharged with an appointment with a therapist to follow up, he managed to abstain from drinking for two months. One problem, however, was that he did not socialize at all with friends during that time. He stayed with his parents and drove to classes for the remainder of that spring semester. He talked to some male friends as well as some female friends via cellphone and Facebook, but otherwise he remained socially isolated. The thought of accepting an invitation to socialize brought on the old anxiety, so he made excuses, including the truth—that he'd decided to quit drinking.

After nearly three months of sobriety, Michael was feeling physically well and energetic but also bored. He gladly helped out around his parents' home and resumed his old hobby of rebuilding old stereo equipment. He chose not to go to AA meetings, however, and his nights were becoming increasingly uncomfortable. Then one day a female friend, Gretchen, whom Michael had something of a crush on, called. She said she'd been told that Michael had decided to stop drinking and that she supported that decision. She added that she had no expectation of his drinking around her and she could also abstain if that would help. Then she said that she was planning a Fourth of July party and she would love it if Michael would come. He replied that he'd think about it and let her know.

The cognitive context of Michael's relapse (and it is a common one) had to do with Michael telling himself that it would be safe for him to go to the party because, for one thing, the girl who invited him said that she understood that he was not drinking, and second, that he had nearly three months of sobriety under his belt. That thinking proved to be Michael's undoing. Here's why:

- Though Michael had been sober nearly three months, he had developed a false sense of confidence that at that point he would be immune to his longstanding habit of heavy drinking to easy his anxiety in social situations. The problem was not in Michael's intentions but rather in the false sense of safety he'd settled into.

- Michael had done little, other than in a couple of brief conversations with his therapist, to address his insecurity and consequent social anxiety. Naturally both re-emerged as soon as he set foot at Gretchen's party.
- Though Gretchen had said she would avoid drinking, she had no control over Michael when a male friend offered him a beer and Michael told himself, "I'll have just one." Through the course of the party, one became six, along with a few shots of tequila in orange juice. When Gretchen asked if he was okay, Michael laughed. "Sure!" he said, though she could see that he was drunk. She ended up driving him home for his safety, where she dropped him off with his parents waiting at the door.

Although the details may differ, the central theme of Michael's slip (and its potential for a full relapse) is a common one. It has to do with the cognitive context of his slip—in other words, what he was thinking. For some reason—and this is the common cognitive thread in many relapses—he had told himself that it would be safe (perhaps because he had three months of sobriety or perhaps because Gretchen was there) for him to have a drink. Of course, once he started drinking he couldn't stop. This is the reality of addiction: one drink is not enough, one cigarette is not enough, one snort of cocaine is not enough, and so on. It can be difficult to accept this reality, as all those who have slipped or relapsed know. Therefore the first step in analyzing any slip is to focus on its cognitive context. What was the recovering person really thinking when the slip occurred? That insight is critical to learning how to avoid future slips and relapses. You might call it dangerous thinking and something to be challenged and avoided.

THE SOCIAL CONTEXT OF SLIPS

Whereas the cognitive context of a slip has to do with what a person was thinking, the social context has to do with where they were and who they were with. In many cases the cognitive and social contexts will overlap, though each also needs to be considered separately. In the case of Michael's slip, this overlap is obvious. Not only did he tell himself he could safely have a drink but also he was with friends who drank, and he was at a party.

There are also instances where the social context is the dominant influence. There are those, for example, who fully accept the fact that they need to abstain from substance use yet who either unintentionally or deliberately find themselves in a situation that supports—or among people who support—the very substance use that the recovering person wants to avoid. One common example, discussed earlier, has to do with family. It's no secret that substance abuse is a problem that runs in families, be that for genetic or social reasons. The bottom line for newly sober individuals, however, is that despite their acceptance of the need to abstain as well as their best intentions, they may find it difficult to avoid certain social situations that include family members who are known substance abusers. Emily is an example.

The youngest of three daughters, Emily was raised by a father who had a strong work ethic and was a good provider but who worked two jobs and was not home a lot and an alcoholic mother whose drinking was never the topic of conversation within the family. Her mother, Emily explained, drank every day, and it was not unusual for Emily to find her passed out in bed when she got home from school. So the girls stepped up and took care of the household. Both parents had siblings, so family gatherings tended to be large. There was typically also a great deal of drinking, and Emily knew (though it too was not talked about) that several family members, including aunts, uncles, and cousins, also had drinking problems.

Emily was one of three daughters. The oldest of Emily's sisters went on to finish only high school due largely to her own drinking then married young and settled into family life while working as a low-wage associate in a large hardware chain. The next daughter in line left home at age eighteen to work full time and attend community college and from there became a dental assistant. She eventually moved to another state, where she lived with another woman.

As for Emily, in some ways you could say that she was the most successful child in that she went to college and then on to graduate school, eventually finding work as a financial adviser for a large firm. Her clients liked her, and over time she'd built a significant and loyal client base that made her job secure. She had not married, but she'd had two relationships, each of which had lasted over two years, but both had ended, one because the man decided to pursue a job opportunity abroad (which Emily felt she could not accommodate, given her own career) and the other when the man proposed marriage and Emily realized that she did not love him that much.

Along the way, Emily, like her mother, gradually became more and more of a drinker to the point where she had an insight that alcohol had become too much a part of her life, and she looked up an alcohol counselor. After an initial assessment the counselor agreed that Emily had progressed to the point of a moderate alcohol-abuse disorder. They discussed moderation, but when Emily talked about her mother the counselor advocated quitting altogether to avoid a repetition of her mother's fate.

Emily also met with her doctor, who supported the decision to abstain and also recommended that Emily start taking Naltrexone, a medication that can help reduce cravings for alcohol. Between her own decision to stop, the support of a counselor, and the medication, Emily was able to achieve abstinence. A year later she was feeling well physically, had lost ten pounds and improved her conditioning by joining a gym, and had started dating a man whom she felt—for the first time—might be someone she'd think about committing to if things progressed in that direction.

Emily had stuck with her therapy, and during that first year of sobriety she pretty much avoided face-to-face contact with her family in favor of phone calls and emails. But then the issue of her parents' fiftieth anniversary came up. Emily's sister felt that they should plan something for everyone. The problem for Emily, though, was that she knew that her mother was not the only family member who drank, and she was sure that there was bound to be ample alcohol at any anniversary celebration. The question then was what should Emily do about the party?

Emily's dilemma is a typical example of a social context that can contribute to a possible slip or relapse. There are certainly people who intentionally place themselves in such risky situations, even with the intent of staying clean and sober, thinking that they will be safe. Too often this proves to be a false hope. In Emily's case, though, she had the advantage of knowing in advance that in this risky situation, her safety wouldn't be assured. On the one hand, she was confident in her sobriety and committed to it; on the other hand, she knew full well that she was in recovery from an alcohol-abuse disorder and remained vulnerable to situations that could tempt her resolve. She did not have a close loved one who could step into the role of collaborator in her recovery, but she did have a therapist she felt close to and trusted. Emily and her therapist decided together that Emily had three choices: go to the party and risk drinking; go to the party, not drink, and be uncomfortable the whole time; or not go. In the end they agreed that the best course for her was to tell both sisters that she was in recovery from a drinking problem, had done well for over a year, and although she would send an anniversary gift to her parents, she would not be attending the celebration. This was, to be sure, a brave decision on Emily's part. She could not be sure how her sisters would react much less what her parents or relatives would think. But the bottom line was that she was willing to risk that as opposed to risking her recovery.

The newly sober and his or her loved ones can use the following as a guide in discussing this issue of the social context of slips:

- As you did in our earlier discussion of risky versus safe places, identify places where your risk of using alcohol or drugs is minimal. These may be, for example, favorite activities (working out, running, playing tennis) or places (museums, shopping malls, restaurants without liquor licenses).
- Take an honest inventory of those social situations that have been associated with your drinking or drug use in the past and ones that are likely to be (e.g., a family birthday or anniversary party).
- Decide what would be the best course of action in such social situations moving forward. Can your loved ones play a role in helping you deal with them?

THE EMOTIONAL CONTEXT OF SLIPS

Thus far we have covered two of the three contexts that are associated with slips and relapses. These are, respectively, "What were you thinking?" and "Who were you with?" To complete our analysis of a slip, we also need to consider a third question: "What were you feeling?" If the newly sober person (along with a loved one) is able to answer these questions, he or she will have a leg up on avoiding a slip or relapse moving forward. To answer the third question, it's important to be able to identify those emotions that are most often associated with alcohol or drug use. We will look at several and discuss why they make individuals vulnerable to substance use that can escalate over time.

Anxiety

Men and women have long turned to alcohol or drugs in an effort to self-medicate anxiety. In low doses (low-risk drinking), alcohol can actually help to reduce anxiety. One glass of wine before a social event can help a shy person overcome his or her social anxiety enough to be able to socialize. As the expression goes, a little alcohol in these situations helps a shy person "come out of their shell." The problem is that for those people whose genetic makeup includes the ability to build a tolerance to alcohol over time, one glass of wine (or one cocktail) can easily progress to two, three, or more. At that point alcohol ceases to have a tranquilizing effect and begins to have a depressive effect. That depression, mild as it may be, can invite more drinking. And so the pathway opens to an alcohol-use disorder. The same cycle applies pretty much as well to cannabis, which in small doses tends to relax but in stronger doses leads to a distancing effect—like viewing the world, as one man said, through a sheer curtain. Tranquilizers operate in much the same fashion and can progress just as alcohol and cannabis can.

Anxiety disorders tend to run in families, as previously discussed, and they may reflect a genetic vulnerability. They can also, however, be part of another disorder, such as PTSD. People who suffer from anxiety may be ashamed to admit it. However, if a newly sober person (along with his or her loved ones) is able to recognize his or her own anxiety disorder and where it comes into play, they can explore other ways of dealing with it. CBT, for example, has been found to be effective in treating social anxiety.[1] With this in mind, the better course of action (as opposed to trying to hide the problem or "treat" it using drugs or alcohol) would be to seek out a therapist with expertise in helping individuals overcome their social anxiety. Failing that, it becomes a real challenge for the anxious individual and his or her loved ones to devise a lifestyle that avoids situations that trigger anxiety.

Depression

It's sometimes said colloquially that people "drown their sorrows" in alcohol. This attests to just how common it is for an individual to turn to drinking (or drugs) to essentially help erase a depression that may hang over them like a cloud. Just as people have long attempted to cope with anxiety by drinking, so have they resorted to alcohol or drugs in an attempt to escape depression. The irony is that alcohol is actually a depressant so that while temporary relief might be found through drinking, in the long run alcohol's perceived benefits will certainly boomerang and worsen the depression.

Here again a collaborative approach may be the best approach. The depressed individual, much like the anxious person, may be reluctant to admit to suffering from depression—or even to recognize the symptoms for what they are. Yet loved ones may have a more accurate perception here. Admitting to depression can be difficult. Its causes can range from lifestyle issues such as a failed relationship to physical issues such as poor health or disability to more existential issues such as a lack of a sense of meaning.

Today the recognized approach to dealing with depression is to combine medication with psychotherapy. Several psychotherapeutic approaches have been studied and found to be helpful in this regard.[2] Either approach alone—medication or psychotherapy—is not likely to be as effective as the two in combination.

Loneliness

There is no quantifiable research on the treatment of loneliness, but one thing we do know is that the number of Americans who are facing the challenge of growing old alone is already staggering and growing.[3] The challenges this population faces include an extended family (children) as well as longstanding friends who are no longer geographically close, plus divorce or widowhood. In addition, there are many who, while not yet seniors, confront isolation and its consequence—loneliness—on a daily basis due to the constraints placed on them by their lifestyle. This may include those who never marry or have children, or those who are single parents who have to work hard to support their children as well as themselves and have precious little time to spare. It can also include those whose occupation requires frequent relocation, leaving them with no time to put down roots.

It isn't hard to understand why individuals in the above situations might turn to drinking or tranquilizers as a means of comfort. Again, at the low-risk level, alcohol can have a comforting effect, and it's been used that way literally for centuries. As with anxiety and depression, however, this use can gradually progress along the substance-use spectrum through a mild disorder all the way to a severe disorder and especially among those men and women who are constitutionally able to build a tolerance to alcohol.

Working through the emotional context of slips and relapses begins, as with the other contexts, with some insight. Readers are wise to devote some time to taking stock of their lifestyle to determine if, indeed, loneliness might be an issue for them. If that turns out to be true, the solution lies not in trying to simply erase loneliness (which is not feasible) but rather to work on making lifestyle changes that replace loneliness and isolation with some sense of social connection. Here are a couple of examples.

Gina, at thirty-four, found herself in what she later called a "lifestyle cage." Having divorced a husband who turned out to be a serial cheater, she had two children whom she was raising without help or child support. Her parents, as much as they loved her and their grandchildren, had retired to another state and were not available for help. She worked as an administrative assistant in a large health insurance firm and was able to support herself and the children, but her job was also demanding and when she returned home from work each day, there her children were, finishing their homework after having been dropped off by bus after school or an after-school activity, and hungry. They shared meal preparation (though the children liked what Gina could make much better) and dinner, after which Gina prepared for the next work day and relaxed by watching TV or reading. A couple of glasses of wine were also a part of her relaxing, but they eventually grew into three, then four glasses of wine every night. She drank her last glass of wine to help her get to sleep, but then she'd wake up in the middle of the night and find it very difficult to get back to sleep. The result was that she felt less and less energetic during the day. She brought this up during her annual physical, suggesting that maybe she needed a sleeping pill, but her doctor was astute and quickly focused on her drinking. The doctor also suggested counseling because it was apparent that Gina was stuck in a lifestyle characterized by isolation, and the doctor told Gina it was easy to see that drinking had become part of that. The solution, the doctor suggested, was not in medication.

Gina's solution took some time to evolve. During that process, though, she was able to severely limit her drinking so as to have more energy. The first change she made in her lifestyle was to get involved in a committee that was devoted to helping guide her town's development. This proved to be a diverse group of people, many married but some single, and it gave Gina a sense of purpose. She also made two new women friends whose lives mirrored her own in many ways. Later she signed up for two workshops through her community's adult education program, one in pottery making and the other in creative writing. In the latter she met a single man, and they spent some time together. Although she did not see this man as a romantic interest, they did share some common interests such as hiking and attending talks offered by the local affiliate of a national outdoor club. Although these changes did not exactly turn Gina's lifestyle upside down, she found that she could pursue these interests without sacrificing her parenting responsibilities (which, to tell the truth, had been a bit excessive because they went back to the years when her children were much younger). A year later, she reported that she no longer felt isolated and that loneliness was also not an emotion she identified with.

Peter, sixty-nine, had retired from his job as an engineer four years earlier. For more than forty years his lifestyle had been that of the main provider for his family and a respected professional at work. His wife, Marie, had retired a year earlier. She had found an outlet as a part-time, in-home daycare provider for their oldest daughter's three-year-old daughter. This required that Marie commute about two hours, so she often spent one or two nights at her daughter's in a spare bedroom. Marie found this very satisfying, particularly as a former primary school teacher. Peter, on the other hand, described his new lifestyle this way: "I watch our two dogs, read books on history, and watch the news." That was it. Aside from having retired from an intellectually challenging job, Peter had at one time had a few good male friends, including two he'd played golf with weekly. Unfortunately, two of them had died and one moved away for retirement in a warmer climate. His contact with the lone remaining friend had gradually fallen by the wayside, though Peter had no good explanation for why.

Like Gina in the above example, Peter found some solace in drinking, although his preference was for martinis rather than wine. Nevertheless, his martini consumption gradually increased to the point where he now typically fell asleep on the couch while watching the news and as early as 8 p.m. That would not have described him in the past.

It was Marie who was responsible for Peter taking the first steps to climb out of the depression and loneliness that he had fallen victim to. Basically she confronted him, saying that it bothered her deeply to see the husband whom she knew to be so intelligent and productive slip into a state she described as "vegetative." Moreover, she said she was beginning to worry about Peter's physical and mental health if he did not do something to help himself.

As it turned out, Peter's longstanding avocation was as a student of history, in particular American history. The first step he took in heeding Marie's advice was to reach out to his one remaining male friend and suggest they meet for lunch. The friend responded that he had missed their former regular contact as well and was happy to meet.

It was during lunch that the friend asked Peter if he'd read any interesting history books lately, as they shared that interest. Peter said he had to admit that he'd pretty much let all of his interests go and that making contact was his first step toward breaking out of his isolation. The friend said he could identify with that and then added that one thing he'd found helpful as well as engaging was to explore some of the online groups that were available and that focused on history. That piqued Peter's interest because he'd never thought of it, and he fired up his computer as soon as he got home that afternoon.

One of the keys to Peter's solution for his situation (in addition to strictly limiting himself to no more that five martinis a week!) was to join several online chat groups that were sponsored by the Smithsonian Institute, each of which focused on a different aspect of American history. Peter found this intellectually stimulating and also a way to connect to others. Soon he was reading voraciously again and sharing his thoughts with others. A few months later he learned through a chat room about an organization in his state that ran a small Civil War museum. He contacted the organization and arranged to volunteer once a month at the museum, helping visitors understand some of the displays.

Boredom

Peter's and Gina's cases illustrate how loneliness and isolation can tempt individuals to turn to substance use as a means of finding solace and comfort. Unfortunately, that solace can also lead to a progression along the substance-use spectrum, and trouble. Another common emotional factor that can play a role in the context of a slip or relapse is boredom. It is particularly a common part of the context of substance abuse in youths.

The term "ennui" refers to the emotional context associated with boredom, and it is defined as "a feeling of listlessness and dissatisfaction arising from a lack of occupation or excitement."[4]

This sense of being adrift, with no clear goal or any articulated values, is an emotional state that youthful substance abusers frequently identify with. It is, understandably, an emotional state that is extremely uncomfortable, and one can easily see how it might invite substance use as a means of escape. Youths are inclined to drink, as are adults, but they are even more inclined to turn to cannabis and prescription drugs such as tranquilizers and psychostimulants that are prescribed for attention-deficit disorder (ADD). It isn't uncommon to find youths using all of these concurrently.

While youths may say that the above definition of "ennui" accurately describes how they feel much of the time, they are typically at a loss for a means to escape it other than getting high. This may describe any newly sober youth reading this book, and his or her loved ones may agree that this seems to describe the youth as well. The issue then becomes, as with the other emotional contexts described above, what is the answer?

The position on boredom and ennui taken here is that the solution lies in exploring spirituality. The link between spirituality and recovery has been discussed (see chapter 10), and it is of particular relevance here. Recall that researchers found that participating in activities they defined as spiritual was associated with improved sobriety and that the reverse was also true: that sustained recovery was associated with increasing involvement in spiritual activities.

If the opposite of ennui lies in a lifestyle that is characterized by "a feeling of meaning and satisfaction deriving from a sense of occupation and excitement," here are some activities that arguably could be said to contribute to this:

- engaging in altruistic activities such as community service and volunteerism—Help others while looking for nothing in return other than a sense of having been useful or comforting.
- connecting with art or nature—Become involved in local conservation efforts; help promote wildlife preservation; go hiking; visit art museums or showings; take a course in creative art or drawing.
- meditating or praying—Practice mindfulness meditation or yoga. Read daily meditations or prayers, and try to implement them in daily life.
- contemplating life goals that can lead to a sense of meaning and purpose—Why am I here? What values do I stand for?

The above constitute only a few suggestions for what spirituality is and how spirituality can play a role in a person's lifestyle. Readers should feel free to brainstorm about them. Newly sober individuals and their loved ones are strongly encouraged to engage in a dialogue about them and to consider how they might go about adding to the spiritual dimension of their lives.

SUMMING UP

If there is a lesson to be learned from this chapter, it is that slips and relapses don't simply fall out of the sky. They are not random events nor do they occur outside of any context. The newly sober person and his or her loved ones can benefit from understanding this context of slips and relapses. Here they are again:

- the cognitive context—What were you thinking?
- the social context—Who were you with?
- the emotional context—What were you feeling?

Armed with this insight, the person who has slipped (or even totally relapsed) and his or her loved ones can work collaboratively to plan ahead so as to minimize such events moving forward.

Epilogue

$\mathcal{T}$his book set out with the goal of providing a guide for the newly sober and their loved ones for building upon and strengthening recovery after rehab or treatment. That recovery can rightly be compared to a voyage across open water. There is no guarantee of success, and obstacles are likely to be encountered along the way. However, with adequate preparation, including knowledge of the potential obstacles and how they can be overcome, the chances of a successful journey increase considerably. In fact, the voyage to a life of sobriety (as compared to attempts to limit or moderate substance use) can transform a person's lifestyle for the better.

Responsibility for the success of the voyage to recovery naturally rests most of all on the shoulders of the newly recovering individual, but his or her loved ones can also play an important role in the process, because by virtue of their connection and commitment to the recovering person, they are also stakeholders in the outcome. For that reason, this book has sought to draw loved ones into the recovery process—to include them as part of the solution. For too long, too many of these loved ones have felt shut out of the recovery process, relegated to the sidelines as it were, with little role to play. Hopefully this book will help to reverse that trend to the benefit of both the newly sober and their loved ones.

Notes

INTRODUCTION

1. Dictionary.com, "Point of departure," 2020, www.dictionary.com/browse /point-of-departure?s=t.

CHAPTER 1: AUSPICIOUS BEGINNINGS

1. National Survey of Substance Abuse Treatment Services, 2020, www .samhsa.gov/data/all-reports.

2. National Institute on Drug Abuse, "Drugs, brains, and behavior: The science of addiction," July 2018, www.drugabuse.gov/publications/principles -drug-addiction-treatment-research-based-guide-third-edition/frequently -asked-questions/how-effective-drug-addiction-treatment.

CHAPTER 2: MEDICATION-ASSISTED TREATMENT (MAT)

1. U.S. Food & Drug Administration, "Information about medication-assisted treatment (MAT)," 2020, www.fda.gov/drugs/information-drug-class /information-about-medication-assisted-treatment-mat.

2. DrugRehab.com, "How much does drug rehab cost?" 2020, www.drug rehab.com/treatment/how-much-does-rehab-cost.

3. T. Kosten & T. George, "The neurobiology of opioid dependence: Implications for treatment," *Science and Practice Perspectives* 1, no. 1 (2002): 13–20.

4. Substance Abuse and Mental Health Services Administration, "Naltrexone," 2020, www.samhsa.gov/medication-assisted-treatment/treatment/naltrexone.

5. H. Kranzler & J. Van Kirk, "Efficacy of naltrexone and acamprosate for alcoholism treatment: A meta-analysis," *Alcoholism: Clinical and Experimental Research* 25 (2001): 1335–41; C. Bouza et al., "Efficacy and safety of naltrexone and acamprosate in the treatment of alcohol dependence: A systematic review," *Addiction* 99 (2004): 811–28.

6. G. Rubio, M.A. Jiménez-Arriero, G. Ponce, & T. Palomo, "Naltrexone versus acamprosate: One year follow-up of alcohol dependence treatment," *Alcohol and Alcoholism* 36, no. 5 (2001): 419–25.

7. E.V. Nunes et al., "Treating opioid dependence with injectable extended-release naltrexone (XR-NTX): Who will respond?" *Journal of Addiction Medicine* 9, no. 3 (2015): 238–43.

8. R.P. Mattick, C. Breen, J. Kimber, & M. Davoli, "Methadone maintenance therapy versus no opioid replacement therapy for opioid dependence," *Cochrane Database of Systematic Reviews* 3 (2009): CD002209.

9. R.P. Schwartz et al., "A randomized controlled trial of interim methadone maintenance," *Archives of General Psychiatry* 63, no. 1 (2006): 102–9.

10. P.J. Fudala et al., "Office-based treatment of opiate addiction with a sublingual-tablet formulation of buprenorphine and naloxone," *New England Journal of Medicine* 349, no. 10 (2003): 949–58.

11. J. Kakko, K.D. Svanborg, M.J. Kreek, & M. Heilig, "1-year retention and social function after buprenorphine-assisted relapse prevention treatment for heroin dependence in Sweden: A randomised, placebo-controlled trial," *Lancet* 361, no. 9358 (2003): 662–68.

CHAPTER 3: HOMECOMING

1. A. Kishline, *Moderate drinking: The moderation management guide for people who want to reduce their drinking* (New York: Crown Trade Paperbacks, 1994).

2. K. Humphreys, "Can targeting nondependent problem drinkers and providing Internet-based services expand access to assistance for alcohol problems: A study of the Moderation Management self-help/mutual aid organization," *Journal of Studies on Alcohol* 62 (2001): 528–32.

3. Alcoholics Anonymous, "Membership survey," 2014, www.aa.org/assets/en_US/p-48_membershipsurvey.pdf.

4. S. Bujarski, S.S. O'Malley, K. Lunny, & L.A. Ray, "The effects of drinking goal on treatment outcome for alcoholism," *Journal of Consulting and Clinical Psychology* 81, no. 1 (2013): 13–22.

5. W.R. Miller, A.L. Leckman, H.D. Delaney, & M. Tinkcom, "Long-term follow-up on behavioral self-control training," *Journal of Studies on Alcohol* 53 (1992): 249–61.

6. National Institutes of Health, National Institute on Drug Abuse, "Marijuana research report: Is marijuana addictive?" 2020, www.drugabuse.gov /publications/research-reports/marijuana/marijuana-addictive.

CHAPTER 4: PREPARING TO MOVE FORWARD

1. Wikipedia, "Enabling," 2020, https://en.wikipedia.org/wiki/Enabling.

2. Wikipedia, "Codependency," 2020, https://en.wikipedia.org/wiki /Codependency.

3. Wikipedia, "Enabling," 2020, https://en.wikipedia.org/wiki/Enabling.

4. American Psychiatric Association, "*DSM-5* fact sheets," 2020, www .psychiatry.org/psychiatrists/practice/dsm/educational-resources/dsm-5-fact -sheets.

5. L. Eigen & D. Rowden, "Section 1: Research—A methodology and current estimate of the number of children of alcoholics in the United States," in *Children of alcoholics: Selected readings*, ed. S. Abbott (Rockville, MD: National Association for Children of Alcoholics, 1996), 1–22.

6. C.A. Schoenborn, "Exposure to alcoholism in the family: United States, 1988," *Advance Data from Vital and Health Statistics* 30, no. 205 (1991): 1–13.

7. H. Hardwood, D. Fountain, & G. Livermore, "The economic costs of alcohol and drug abuse in the United States, 1992," NIH publication no. 98-4327 (Rockville, MD: National Institutes of Health, 1998).

8. Wikipedia, "Enabling," 2020, https://en.wikipedia.org/wiki/Enabling.

9. J.P. Morgan, "What is codependency?" *Journal of Clinical Psychology* 47, no. 5 (1991): 720–29.

10. G.E. Dear, C. Roberts, & L. Lange, *Defining codependency: A thematic analysis of published definitions*, in *Advances in psychology, volume 34*, ed. S. Shohov (New York: Nova Science Publishers, 2004), 189–205.

11. N. Lindley, P. Giordano, & E. Hammer, "Codependency: Predictors and psychometric issues," *Journal of Clinical Psychology* 55, no. 1 (1999): 59–64.

CHAPTER 5: POST-REHAB FELLOWSHIPS
AND HOW THEY HELP

1. Wikipedia, "Individualist," 2020, https://en.wikipedia.org/wiki/Individualism.

2. A. Rosenbaum, "Personal space and American individualism," *Brown Political Review*, October 31, 2018, http://brownpoliticalreview.org/2018/10/personal-space-american-individualism.

3. R.H. Moos & B.S. Moos, "Paths of entry into Alcoholics Anonymous: Consequences for participation and remission," *Alcoholism: Clinical and Experimental Research* 29, no. 10 (2005): 1858–68.

4. L.A. Kaskutas et al. *Alcoholics anonymous careers: Patterns of AA involvement five years after treatment entry, Alcoholism: Clinical and Experimental Research* 29, no. 11 (2005): 1983–90.

5. J. Witbrodt et al., "Alcohol and drug treatment involvement: 12-step attendance and abstinence, 9-year cross-lagged analysis of adults in an integrated health plan," *Journal of Substance Abuse Treatment* 46 (2014): 412–19.

6. J.F. Kelly, K. Humphreys, & M. Ferri, "Alcoholics Anonymous and other 12-step programs for alcohol use disorder," 2020, www.cochranelibrary.com/cdsr/doi/10.1002/14651858.CD012880.pub2/full.

7. Alcoholics Anonymous, "Twelve Steps and Twelve Traditions," 2020, www.aa.org/pages/en_US/twelve-steps-and-twelve-traditions.

8. Alcoholics Anonymous, "The A.A. member—Medications & other drugs," 2018, www.aa.org/assets/en_US/p-11_aamembersMedDrug.pdf.

9. First Nations Pedagogy Online, 2020, https://firstnationspedagogy.ca/circletalks.html.

10. Alcoholics Anonymous, "Membership survey," 2014, www.aa.org/assets/en_US/p-48_membershipsurvey.pdf.

11. J.S. Tonigan & S.L. Rice, "Is it beneficial to have an Alcoholics Anonymous sponsor?" *Psychology of Addictive Behaviors* 24, no. 3 (2010): 397–403.

12. SMART Recovery, "About SMART Recovery," 2020, www.smartrecovery.org/about-us.

13. SMART Recovery.

14. SMART Recovery.

15. SMART Recovery Training, "GSF 201: Facilitator training," 2020, https://smartrecoverytraining.org/Library/Docs/Syllabus_GSF201.pdf.

16. A.K. Beck et al., "Systematic review of SMART Recovery: Outcomes, process variables, and implications for research," *Psychology of Addictive Behaviors* 31, no. 1 (2017): 1–20, doi:10.1037/adb0000237.

17. P. Guth, "Jean Kirkpatrick author brings hope to women alcoholics," *Morning Call*, April 13, 1995 https://www.mcall.com/news/mc-xpm-1995-04 -13-3040809-story.html.
18. Women for Sobriety, "New Life Program," 2020, https://womenfor sobriety.org/new-life-program/.
19. Women for Sobriety, "WFS New Life Program Acceptance Statements," https://womenforsobriety.org/wp-content/uploads/2018/01/WFS_New _Life_Acceptance_Statements.pdf.
20. S. Cahalan, "Baldwin: I was an Alec-oholic," *New York Post*, January 11, 2009, https://nypost.com/2009/01/11/baldwin-i-was-an-alec-oholic.

CHAPTER 6: CREATING A RECOVERY LIFESTYLE: PART 1

1. S.A. Brown, P. Vick, & V. Creamer, "Characteristics of relapse following adolescent substance abuse treatment," *Addictive Behaviors* 14, no. 3 (1989): 291–300.
2. M.D. Litt, R.M. Kadden, E. Kabela-Cormier, & N.M. Petry, "Changing network support for drinking: Network Support Project 2-year follow-up," *Journal of Consulting and Clinical Psychology* 77, no. 2 (2009): 229–42.

CHAPTER 7: CREATING A RECOVERY LIFESTYLE: PART 2

1. Office of Disease Prevention and Health Promotion, "Appendix 9. Alcohol," 2020, https://health.gov/our-work/food-nutrition/2015-2020-dietary -guidelines/guidelines/appendix-9.
2. American Cancer Society, "Alcohol use and cancer," 2020, www.cancer .org/cancer/cancer-causes/diet-physical-activity/alcohol-use-and-cancer.html.
3. National Center for Biotechnology Information, 2020, www.ncbi.nlm .nih.gov/pmc/articles/PMC4941786; J. Kabat-Zinn, *Full catastrophe living* (New York: Bantam, 2013).

CHAPTER 8: DOUBLE TROUBLE

1. I.L. Petrakis, G. Gonzalez, R. Rosenheck, & J.H. Krystal, "Comorbidity of alcoholism and psychiatric disorders," 2002, http://pubs.niaaa.nih.gov /publications/arh26-2/81-89.htm.

2. Bill W. "A Letter from Bill W. on Depression," Silkworth.net, 1958, https://silkworth.net/alcoholics-anonymous/a-letter-from-bill-w-on-depression.

3. C.A. Prescott, "Sex differences in the genetic risk for alcoholism," National Institutes of Health, National Institute on Alcohol Abuse and Alcoholism, 2003, https://pubs.niaaa.nih.gov/publications/arh26-4/264-273.htm.

4. N.S. Cotton, "The familial incidence of alcoholism: A review," *Journal of Studies on Alcohol* 40 (1979): 89–116.

5. Prescott, "Sex differences."

6. F.W. Lohoff, "Overview of the genetics of major depressive disorder," National Center for Biotechnology Information, 2010, www.ncbi.nlm.nih.gov /pmc/articles/PMC3077049; D.F. Levinson, "The genetics of depression: A review," *Biological Psychiatry* 60 (2006): 84–92.

7. R.R. Crowe, "The genetics of panic disorder and agoraphobia," *Psychiatric Developments* 3, no. 2 (1985): 171–85.

8. S. Glassner-Edwards et al., "Mechanisms of action in integrated cognitive-behavioral treatment versus twelve-step facilitation for substance-dependent adults with comorbid major depression," *Journal of Studies on Alcohol and Drugs* 68 (2007): 663–72.

9. E. Triffleman, "Gender differences in a controlled pilot study of psychosocial treatments in substance dependent patients with post-traumatic stress disorder: Design considerations and outcomes," *Alcoholism Treatment Quarterly* 18, no. 3 (2000): 113–26.

10. J. Nowinski & S. Baker, *The Twelve Step facilitation handbook, second edition* (Center City, MN: Hazelden Publications, 2017).

CHAPTER 9: HEALING DAMAGED RELATIONSHIPS

1. H.M. Tiebout, "Ego factors in surrender in alcoholism," *Quarterly Journal of Studies on Alcohol* (1954): 610–21.

2. F. Zeidan and D. Vago, "Mindfulness meditation–based pain relief: A mechanistic account," National Center for Biotechnology Information, 2016, www.ncbi.nlm.nih.gov/pmc/articles/PMC4941786.

CHAPTER 10: SPIRITUALITY AND RECOVERY

1. S. Carroll, "Spirituality and purpose in life in alcoholism recovery," *Journal of Studies on Alcoholism* 54 (1993): 297–301.

2. J.F. Kelly et al., "Spirituality in recovery: A lagged mediational analysis of Alcoholics Anonymous' principal theoretical mechanism of behavior change," *Alcoholism: Clinical and Experimental Research* 35, no. 3 (2011): 454–63.

3. G.J. Connors, J.S. Tonigan, & W.R. Miller, "A measure of religious background and behavior for use in behavior change research," *Psychology of Addictive Behaviors* 10, no. 2 (1996): 90–96.

CHAPTER 11: WHAT IF IT DOESN'T WORK?

1 B.O. Olatunji, J.M. Cisler, & B.J. Deacon, "Efficacy of cognitive behavioral therapy for anxiety disorders: A review of meta-analytic findings," *Psychiatric Clinics of North America* 33, no. 3 (2010): 557–77.

2. P. Cuijpers, A. van Straten, G. Andersson, & P. van Oppen, "Psychotherapy for depression in adults: A meta-analysis of comparative outcome studies," *Journal of Consulting and Clinical Psychology* 76, no. 6 (2008): 909–22.

3. U.S. Congress Joint Economic Committee, "An invisible tsunami: 'Aging alone' and its effect on older Americans, families, and taxpayers," 2019, www .jec.senate.gov/public/index.cfm/republicans/2019/1/an-invisible-tsunami -lsquo-aging-alone-rsquo-and-its-impact-on-older-americans-families-and -taxpayers.

4. Lexico.com, "Definition of *Ennui* in English," 2020, www.lexico.com /en/definition/ennui.

Bibliography

Alcoholics Anonymous. "Membership survey." 2014. www.aa.org/assets/en_US /p-48_membershipsurvey.pdf.
———. "The A.A. member—Medications & other drugs." 2018. www.aa.org /assets/en_US/p-11_aamembersMedDrug.pdf.
———. "Twelve Steps and Twelve Traditions." 2020. www.aa.org/pages /en_US/twelve-steps-and-twelve-traditions.
American Cancer Society. "Alcohol use and cancer." 2020. www.cancer.org /cancer/cancer-causes/diet-physical-activity/alcohol-use-and-cancer.html.
American Psychiatric Association. "DSM-5 fact sheets." 2020. www.psychiatry .org/psychiatrists/practice/dsm/educational-resources/dsm-5-fact-sheets.
Beck, A.K., E. Forbes, A.L. Baker, P.J. Kelly, P. Deane, A. Shakeshaft, D. Hunt, & J.F. Kelly. "Systematic review of SMART Recovery: Outcomes, process variables, and implications for research." *Psychology of Addictive Behaviors* 31, no. 1 (2017): 1–20. doi:10.1037/adb0000237.
Bouza, C., M. Angeles, A. Muñoz, & J.M. Amate. "Efficacy and safety of naltrexone and acamprosate in the treatment of alcohol dependence: A systematic review." *Addiction* 99 (2004): 811–28.
Brown, S.A., P. Vick, & V. Creamer. "Characteristics of relapse following adolescent substance abuse treatment." *Addictive Behaviors* 14, no. 3 (1989): 291–300.
Bujarski, S., S.S. O'Malley, K. Lunny, & L.A. Ray. "The effects of drinking goal on treatment outcome for alcoholism." *Journal of Consulting and Clinical Psychology* 81, no. 1 (2013): 13–22.
Connors, G.J., J.S. Tonigan, & W.R. Miller. "A measure of religious background and behavior for use in behavior change research." *Psychology of Addictive Behaviors* 10, no. 2 (1996): 90–96.
Cotton, N.S. "The familial incidence of alcoholism: A review." *Journal of Studies on Alcohol* 40 (1979): 89–116.

Crowe, R.R. "The genetics of panic disorder and agoraphobia." *Psychiatric Developments* 3, no. 2 (1985): 171–85.

Cuijpers, P., A. van Straten, G. Andersson, & P. van Oppen. "Psychotherapy for depression in adults: A meta-analysis of comparative outcome studies." *Journal of Consulting and Clinical Psychology* 76, no. 6 (2008): 909–22.

Dear, G.E., C. Roberts, & L. Lange. Defining codependency: A thematic analysis of published definitions. In *Advances in Psychology*, edited by S. Shohov, 34 (2004): 189—205. New York: Nova Science Publishers.

DrugRehab.com. "How much does drug rehab cost?" 2020. www.drugrehab .com/treatment/how-much-does-rehab-cost.

Eigen, L., & D. Rowden. "Section 1: Research—A methodology and current estimate of the number of children of alcoholics in the United States." In *Children of alcoholics: Selected readings* edited by S. Abbott, Rockville, MD: National Association for Children of Alcoholics. 1–22.

First Nations Pedagogy Online. 2020. https://firstnationspedagogy.ca/circle talks.html.

Fudala, P.J., T.P. Bridge, S. Herbert, W.O. Williford, C.N. Chiang, K. Jones, J. Collins, D. Raisch, P. Casadonte, R.J. Goldsmith, W. Ling, U. Malkerneker, L. McNicholas, J. Renner, S. Stine, & D. Tusel. "Office-based treatment of opiate addiction with a sublingual-tablet formulation of buprenorphine and naloxone." *New England Journal of Medicine* 349, no. 10 (2003): 949–58.

Glassner-Edwards, S., S.R. Tate, J.R. McQuaid, K. Cummins, E. Granholm, & S.A. Brown. "Mechanisms of action in integrated cognitive-behavioral treatment versus twelve-step facilitation for substance-dependent adults with comorbid major depression." *Journal of Studies on Alcohol and Drugs* 68 (2007): 663–72.

Hardwood, H., D. Fountain, & G. Livermore. "The economic costs of alcohol and drug abuse in the United States, 1992." NIH publication no. 98-4327. Rockville, MD: National Institutes of Health, 1998.

Humphreys, K. "Can targeting nondependent problem drinkers and providing internet-based services expand access to assistance for alcohol problems: A study of the moderation management self-help/mutual aid organization." *Quarterly Journal of Studies on Alcohol* 62 (2001): 528–32.

Kabat-Zinn, J. *Full catastrophe living*. New York: Bantam, 2013.

Kakko J., K.D. Svanborg, M.J. Kreek, & M. Heilig. "1-year retention and social function after buprenorphine-assisted relapse prevention treatment for heroin dependence in Sweden: A randomised, placebo-controlled trial." *Lancet* 361, no. 9358 (2003): 662–68.

Kaskutas, L.A., L. Ammon, K. Delucchi, R. Room, J. Bond, & C. Weisner. "Alcoholics Anonymous careers: Patterns of AA involvement five years after treatment entry." *Alcoholism: Clinical and Experimental Research* 29, no. 11 (2005): 1983–90.

Kelly, J.F., K. Humphreys, & M. Ferri. "Alcoholics Anonymous and other 12-step programs for alcohol use disorder." 2020. www.cochranelibrary.com /cdsr/doi/10.1002/14651858.CD012880.pub2/full.

Kelly, J.F., R.L. Stout, M. Magill, J.S. Tonigan, & M.E. Pagano. "Spirituality in recovery: A lagged mediational analysis of Alcoholics Anonymous' principal theoretical mechanism of behavior change." *Alcoholism: Clinical and Experimental Research* 35, no. 3 (2011): 454–63.

Kishline, A. *Moderate drinking: The moderation management guide for people who want to reduce their drinking.* New York: Crown Trade Paperbacks, 1994.

Kosten, T., & T. George. "The neurobiology of opioid dependence: Implications for treatment." *Science and Practice Perspectives* 1, no. 1 (2002): 13–20.

Kranzler, H., & J. Van Kirk. "Efficacy of naltrexone and acamprosate for alcoholism treatment: A meta-analysis." *Alcoholism: Clinical and Experimental Research* 25 (2001): 1335–41.

Levinson, D.F. "The genetics of depression: A review." *Biological Psychiatry* 60 (2006): 84–92.

Lindley, N., P. Giordano, & E. Hammer. "Codependency: Predictors and psychometric issues." *Journal of Clinical Psychology* 55, no. 1 (1999): 59–64.

Litt, M.D., R.M. Kadden, E. Kabela-Cormier, & N.M. Petry. "Changing network support for drinking: Network Support Project 2-year follow-up." *Journal of Consulting and Clinical Psychology* 77, no. 2 (2009): 229–42.

Lohoff, F.W. "Overview of the genetics of major depressive disorder." National Center for Biotechnology Information. 2010. www.ncbi.nlm.nih.gov/pmc /articles/PMC3077049.

Mattick, R.P., C. Breen, J. Kimber, & M. Davoli. "Methadone maintenance therapy versus no opioid replacement therapy for opioid dependence." *Cochrane Database of Systematic Reviews* 3 (2009): CD002209.

Miller, W.R., A.L. Leckman, H.D. Delaney, & M. Tinkcom. "Long-term follow-up on behavioral self-control training." *Journal of Studies on Alcohol* 53 (1992): 249–61.

Moos, R.H., & B.S. Moos. "Paths of entry into Alcoholics Anonymous: Consequences for participation and remission." *Alcoholism: Clinical and Experimental Research* 29, no. 10 (2005): 1858–68.

Morgan, J.P. "What is codependency?" *Journal of Clinical Psychology* 47, no. 5 (1991): 720–29.

National Institutes of Health, National Institute on Drug Abuse. "Drugs, brains, and behavior: The science of addiction." 2018. www.drugabuse.gov /publications/principles-drug-addiction-treatment-research-based-guide -third-edition/frequently-asked-questions/how-effective-drug-addiction -treatment.

————. "Marijuana research report: Is marijuana addictive?" 2020. www.drug abuse.gov/publications/research-reports/marijuana/marijuana-addictive.

National Survey of Substance Abuse Treatment Services. 2020. www.samhsa .gov/data/all-reports.

Nunes, E.V., E. Krupitsk, W. Ling, J. Zummo, A. Memisoglu, B.L. Silverman, & D. Gastfriend. "Treating opioid dependence with injectable extended-release naltrexone (XR-NTX): Who will respond?" *Journal of Addiction Medicine* 9, no. 3 (2015): 238–43.

Office of Disease Prevention and Health Promotion. "Appendix 9. Alcohol." 2020. https://health.gov/our-work/food-nutrition/2015-2020-dietary -guidelines/guidelines/appendix-9.

Olatunji, B.O., J.M. Cisler, & B.J. Deacon. "Efficacy of cognitive behavioral therapy for anxiety disorders: A review of meta-Analytic findings." *Psychiatric Clinics of North America* 33, no. 3 (2010): 557–77.

Petrakis, I.L., G. Gonzalez, R. Rosenheck, & J.H. Krystal. "Comorbidity of alcoholism and psychiatric disorders." 2002. http://pubs.niaaa.nih.gov/pub lications/arh26-2/81-89.htm.

Prescott, C.A. "Sex differences in the genetic risk for alcoholism." National Institutes of Health, National Institute on Alcohol Abuse and Alcoholism. 2003. https://pubs.niaaa.nih.gov/publications/arh26-4/264-273.htm.

Rosenbaum, A. "Personal space and American individualism." *Brown Political Review*. 2018. https://brownpoliticalreview.org/2018/10/personal-space -american-individualism/.

Rubio G., M.A. Jiménez-Arriero, G. Ponce, & T. Palomo. "Naltrexone versus acamprosate: One year follow-up of alcohol dependence treatment." *Alcohol and Alcoholism* 36, no. 5 (2001): 419–25.

Schoenborn, C.A. "Exposure to alcoholism in the family: United States, 1988." *Advance Data from Vital and Health Statistics* 30, no. 205 (1991): 1–13.

Schwartz, R.P., D.A. Highfield, J.H. Jaffe, J.V. Brady, C.B. Butler, C.O. Rouse, J.M. Callaman, K.E. O'Grady, & R.J. Battjes. "A randomized controlled trial of interim methadone maintenance." *Archives of General Psychiatry* 63, no. 1 (2006): 102–9.

SMART Recovery. "About SMART Recovery." 2020. www.smartrecovery .org/about-us.

SMART Recovery Training. "GSF 201: Facilitator training." 2020. https:// smartrecoverytraining.org/Library/Docs/Syllabus_GSF201.pdf.

Substance Abuse and Mental Health Services Administration. "Naltrexone." 2020. www.samhsa.gov/medication-assisted-treatment/treatment/naltrexone.

Tiebout, H.M. "Ego factors in surrender in alcoholism." *Quarterly Journal of Studies on Alcohol* (1954): 610–21.

Tonigan, J.S., & S.L. Rice. "Is it beneficial to have an Alcoholics Anonymous sponsor?" *Psychology of Addictive Behaviors* 24, no. 3 (2010): 397–403.

U.S. Congress Joint Economic Committee. "An invisible tsunami: 'Aging alone' and its effect on older Americans, families, and taxpayers." 2019. www.jec.senate.gov/public/index.cfm/republicans/2019/1/an-invisible-tsu nami-lsquo-aging-alone-rsquo-and-its-impact-on-older-americans-fami lies-and-taxpayers.

U.S. Food & Drug Administration. "Information about medication-assisted treatment (MAT)." 2020. www.fda.gov/drugs/information-drug-class/in formation-about-medication-assisted-treatment-mat.

Volkow, N.D. "How science has revolutionized the understanding of drug addiction." 2020. National Institutes of Health, National Institute on Drug Abuse. www.drugabuse.gov/publications/drugs-brains-behavior-science -addiction/preface.

Witbrodt, J., M.A. Yu Ye, J. Bond, F. Chi, C. Weisner, & J. Mertens. "Alcohol and drug treatment involvement: 12-step attendance and abstinence, 9-year cross-lagged analysis of adults in an integrated health plan." *Journal of Substance Abuse Treatment* 46 (2014): 412–19.

Women for Sobriety. "New Life Program." 2020. https://womenforsobriety .org/new-life-program/.

Zeidan, F., & D. Vago. "Mindfulness meditation–based pain relief: A mechanistic account." National Center for Biotechnology Information. 2016. www.ncbi.nlm.nih.gov/pmc/articles/PMC4941786.

Index

psychotherapy, 29; for co-occurring
disorders, 96; for depression, 134
PTSD. *See* post-traumatic stress
disorder

radical individualism, 41–42
RBB. *See* Religious Background and
Behavior questionnaire
reading spiritual materials, 117, 119
recovery fellowships, 72; AA as,
42–53, 61; choice of, 57–59;
combining with treatment
program, 44; involvement, for
recovery, 48; overview, 41–42;
radical individualism and, 41–42;
research, 42–49; SMART
Recovery as, 53–55, 61; WFS as,
55–57, 61
recovery lifestyle: alcohol or drugs
in, 61–64; building social
network for, 65–74; overview,
61; people who support, 72–73;
transformation in, 65
recovery lifestyle, places and routines
in: activities and, 83–87; activities
worksheet for, *84*; limitations in,
81; loved ones included in, 79–82;
overview, 75–79; plan for, 78–79;
pursuit of transformation in, 87;
recovery support associations,
82; risky and safe places, 132;
substance use associations, 82;
substitutions in, 81–82; think
outside box for, 83; working with
therapist, 79; worksheet for, *82,*
83
regression, 102–3; addiction and,
101, 104; in substance use
spectrum, 108. *See also* relapse;
slips and relapses

rehab: compared to sails of schooner,
8, *9*; moving forward, 47;
opaqueness of industry, 3–4;
as point of transformation,
65; recovery beyond, 113;
relationships after, 2; therapy
groups in, 128; 28-day stays in,
7, 65
relapse, 10, 14; depression and,
15; DTR, 23–24; enabling
and, 38; percentages, 4–5;
prescription drugs and, 86; radical
individualism and, 41; social
network and, 68–69, 71. *See also*
slips and relapses
relationships, 27, 56; alcoholism
and, 102, 106; parent-child,
101; serious relationship stage
of substance use, 62–64; with
substance use, 2
relationships, healing damaged:
gradual development in, 110;
listening and, 106–8; open
communication with family
rituals, 110–13; overview, 101–4;
shared goals in, 108–13; substance
abuse and damaged attachments,
104–6
Religious Background and Behavior
questionnaire (RBB), 118–19
religious services, 117, 119; for
reconnecting to religion, 123
research: on AA, 45–47, 52–53,
116–17; on alcohol abuse,
89–90; on controlled use, 22–26,
126; longitudinal study, 44;
on methadone, 11; on MM,
21–22, 126; on PTSD, 98–99;
on recovery fellowships, 42–49;
SMART Recovery and, 54–55;
on sobriety, 96–99; on social

of mental illness, 93; genetics of substance abuse, 92–93; moving forward, 99; self-medication and, 91–92; treatment for co-occurring disorders, 95–99
substance dependency post-traumatic stress disorder therapy (SDPT), 98–99
substance use: casual friendship stage, 62; commitment stage, 64; medical issues from, 64; people who support, 70–72; places and routines associated with, 82; in recovery lifestyle, 61–64; relationships with, 2; scale of, 126; serious relationship stage, 62–64
substance use spectrum, 26–27, *27*, 35, 61–62; lifestyle shrinking along, 83, 101; progression along, 138; regression in, 108; social networks in, 69–70
Sunday family dinners, 111–12

tennis, 132
Third Tradition of Alcoholic Anonymous, 50
Tiebout, Harry, 102
Tonigan, J. Scott, 118
tranquilizers, 72, 76, 105, 107, 133, 135, 138

transformation: experience of, 87; in recovery lifestyle, 65
Triffleman, Elisa, 98
Twelve-Step facilitation (TSF), 23, 48, 50; participation in, 98; research findings, 97–99

University of California, Los Angeles, 23, 45
University of New Mexico, 118

VA healthcare system, 97
Vivitrol, 9–10

websites: AA, 50; MM, 21; secular AA, 50; SMART Recovery, 53–54; WFS, 55
wildlife preservation, 139
Wilson, Bill, 50, 55, 92, 102
Women for Sobriety (WFS), 67, 73; abstinence and, 55–56; Acceptance Statements, 56–57; founding of, 55; Levels of Recovery, 56; meetings, 57; recommendations for, 96; as recovery fellowship, 55–57, 61; spirituality and, 120; website, 55
working out, 132

Yale University School of Medicine, 23, 98
yoga, 139

About the Author

Joseph Nowinski, PhD, is an internationally recognized clinical psychologist. He has published several books on the subject of substance abuse, addiction, and recovery and has held positions as assistant professor of psychiatry at the University of California San Francisco School of Medicine, associate professor of psychology at the University of Connecticut, and supervising psychologist at the University of Connecticut Health Center. He currently is an assistant professor at the Hazelden Betty Ford Graduate School of Addiction Studies. For additional information, visit www.josephnowinski.com.